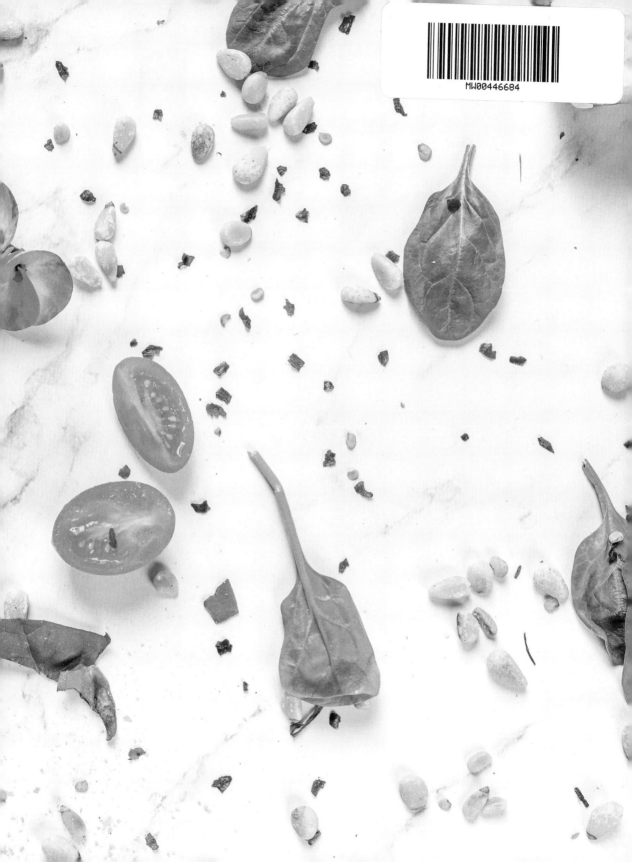

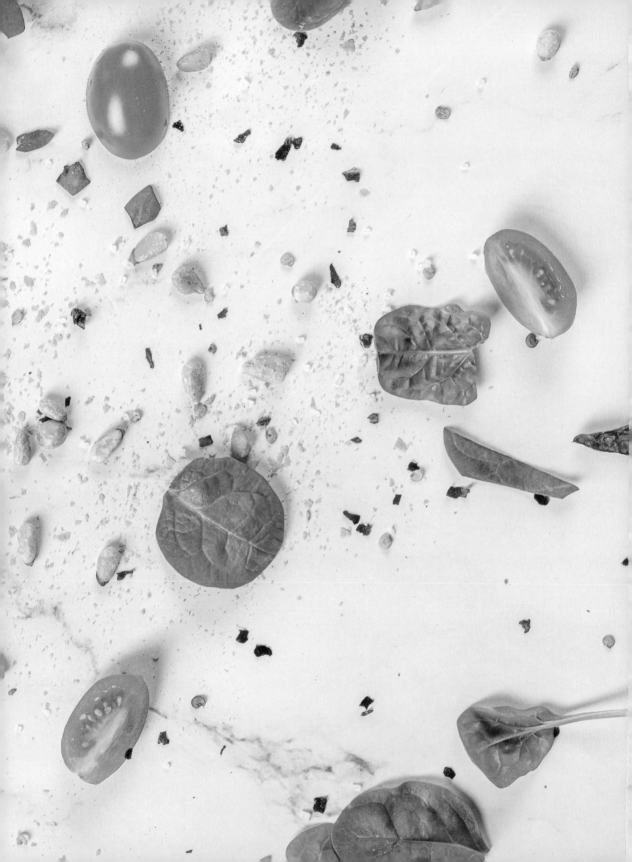

The Type 2 Diabetes Revolution

A Cookbook and Complete Guide to Managing Type 2 Diabetes

By Diana Licalzi, MS, RD, CDCES and Jose Tejero

Dedication

To the millions of people struggling with pre- and type 2 diabetes.

And to our wonderful community, we thank you for your unwavering support, invaluable feedback, and trust in us—all of which made this book possible.

Foreword

Opening and flipping through the pages of a new cookbook is always thrilling. The colorful pictures of delicious meals practically jump off the pages, stimulating your appetite and capturing your interest. The excitement builds as you read the ingredients—some familiar and some new—and as you flip through the recipes and earmark the ones you want to try first.

This cookbook will most certainly have this effect on you *and more*. You see, this is much more than just another cookbook. It is also a tool to help you actively transform your type 2 diabetes, one recipe at a time. The intentional design and selection of recipes in this book will awaken your taste buds and help promote your path to a healthier lifestyle.

Diana Licalzi, a registered dietitian and certified diabetes care and education specialist, and Jose Tejero, an exercise physiologist, are both passionate diabetes experts and professionals dedicated to helping individuals with insulin resistance and type 2 diabetes. They have created this cookbook as a comprehensive resource to guide you toward pushing your type 2 diabetes into remission. Yes, you read that correctly—remission. Did you know that it is possible to reverse the course of type 2 diabetes and put it into remission? It is absolutely true. With this cookbook, you are ready to become a part of this type 2 diabetes revolution.

Type 2 diabetes stems from progressive insulin resistance that has been at play for years. In fact, insulin resistance occurs way before blood sugars begin to rise. Nutrition plays a crucial role in its development, particularly through consistent overconsumption of sugar-sweetened foods high in saturated fat, low in fiber, and rich in ultra-refined carbohydrates. It's important to note that the key factor lies in the consistency with which this unhealthy eating pattern is adopted. No one meal consumed at any one point will cause disease. However, the progressive pattern of unhealthy eating behaviors does contribute to insulin resistance and can progress into overt disease, type 2 diabetes being one such example. So understanding which healthy food combinations and meals can reverse this process allows for an individual to repair the disordered physiology within them that is at play in causing disease. But explaining this crucial detail is frequently left out of the discussion at the time of a diagnosis of type 2 diabetes.

Diana and Jose have been leveraging the notion that knowledge is power and passionately presenting evidence-based approaches to adopting lifestyle changes *first* to prevent or reverse disease course. They have empowered individuals to use nutrition in ways that address the underlying cause of insulin resistance and as a result they have countless stories of individuals who have been able to push their diabetes into remission. Just taking a minute to look at the wonderful content they present on their social media pages will have you extending that minute into hours, as their recommendations are pertinent, accessible, inspiring, and they provide specific evidence-based examples that take the guess work out and set each individual up for success with type 2 diabetes. Want to know protein-rich plant-based snacks? Diana's got that covered. Want to know why fiber is important for blood sugar control? Listen to Jose give an easy to understand, yet in-depth dive into precisely that. And you want to see some mouthwatering meals? There are plenty of examples that have you adding the post to your favorites tab!

And with this cookbook they are now contributing another valuable resource to those who are in search of using food as medicine. This revolutionary cookbook not only magnificently breaks down the complicated physiology of insulin resistance into a way that is easy to digest (pun intended), but also delivers delicious and nutritious recipes that provide you with the tools to reverse insulin resistance via each healthy recipe presented. And here is one of the greatest surprises of all. Healthy eating and *delicious* eating do not have to be mutually exclusive!

I can't wait to share this cookbook with my patients who are looking for assistance in revolutionizing their type 2 diabetes. Their recipes will certainly be on frequent rotation in my teaching kitchen. So, what are we waiting for?! Let's dig in!

Sandra Indacochea Sobel, MD
Endocrinologist
Lifestyle Medicine Specialist
Obesity Medicine Specialist
Founder and CEO, Summon Health

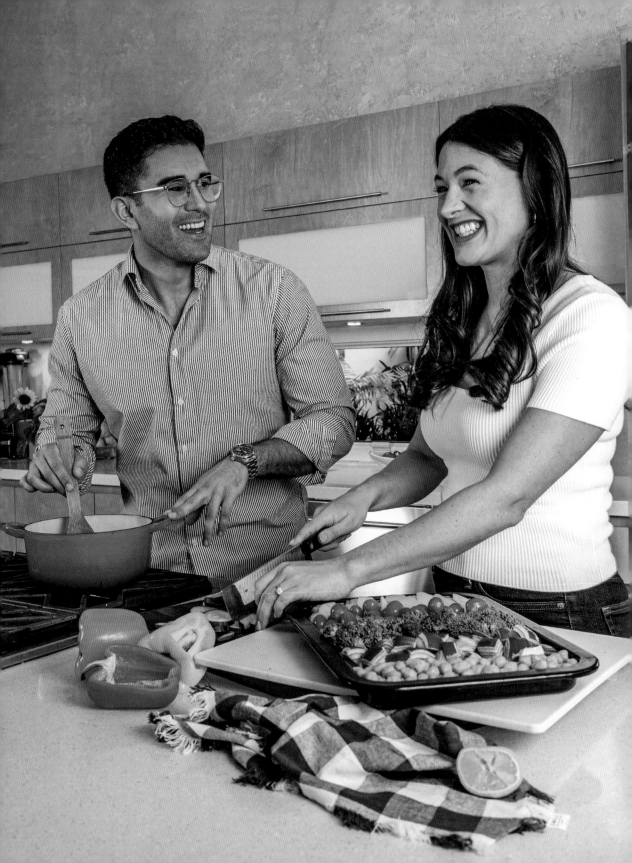

Introduction

If you've picked up this book, there's a good chance you've been recently diagnosed with type 2 diabetes. Or perhaps you've been struggling with this condition for years. Either way, you're not alone. Type 2 diabetes affects 537 million people globally, and is expected to rise to 643 million by 2030. In the United States, more than one-third of the population has pre- or type 2 diabetes, making it the eighth leading cause of death and number one cause of kidney failure, lower-limb amputations, and adult blindness. While diabetes can be a worrying, life-altering condition, you should know that a few tweeks to your diet and lifestyle have the potential to reverse insulin resistance (the root cause of type 2 diabetes), place diabetes into remission, and keep it there. That's where we come in.

Who We Are

We're Diana and Jose, two diabetes experts with over twelve years of combined diabetes work experience.

Diana is a nationally-recognized Registered Dietitian and Certified Diabetes Care and Education Specialist, and holds a Master's in Nutrition Science and Policy. Her journey toward diabetes care began while growing up in Puerto Rico, where she witnessed many of her family members struggling with the condition. After discovering she had a strong genetic predisposition to developing type 2 diabetes, Diana began studying nutrition and its connection to diabetes.

In addition to her Master's from Tufts Friedman School of Nutrition, Diana holds a Didactic Certification in Dietetics from Simmons College. She completed her clinically-focused supervised practice in several different fields within nutrition, including diabetes, cardiology, and oncology, during her Dietetic Internship at UC San Diego Health. After passing the Registered Dietitian national exam, Diana gained experience in various settings, including at Boston Medical Center, Labcorp, and InsideTracker. She worked alongside endocrinologists, dietitians, and other diabetes professionals, eventually fulfilling the requirements to become a Certified Diabetes Care and Education Specialist (CDCES). While working in the healthcare system, Diana grew frustrated by the lack of proper care and education given to people with type 2 diabetes, so she pivoted her focus and started her own private practice dedicated to providing direct, personalized care for this underserved group.

Now on to Jose. Jose is an Exercise Physiologist and holds a Bachelor's degree in Exercise Science from the University of Maryland. Jose initially set out to become a physician, taking pre-med courses and working with two physicians who used plant-based nutrition to heal chronic illnesses, including type 2 diabetes. He saw patients reverse metabolic conditions by merely modifying their diet to a more plant-based one, and was left utterly speechless after observing one patient's HbA1c of 16% drop to 7% in less than three months (more on what this means later!).

Unfortunately, the large majority of patients don't adopt lifestyle changes, in part because time constraints during a typical doctor's visit often prevent this essential discussion. Realizing that he wanted to focus more on exercise and lifestyle, rather than medications, as a way to control diseases, Jose re-evaluated his career path, switched his major to Exercise Science, and graduated as an Exercise Physiologist. However, his interest in plant-based nutrition persisted. After college, he worked at Mastering Diabetes for many years, where he gained a deeper understanding of how to use exercise and a plant-predominant diet to treat diabetes.

Throughout the years, Jose has channeled his passion for exercise into endurance training, completing several half and full marathons, triathlons, and a full Ironman Triathlon—a race consisting of a 2.4-mile (3.9km) swim, a 112-mile (180.2km) bike ride, and a 26.2-mile (42.2km) run.

In 2019, Diana and Jose met through social media and quickly realized how much their mission and goals aligned—both wanted to encourage people with type 2 diabetes to use diet, exercise, and other lifestyle modifications to combat the condition. This is how Reversing T2D was formed. Together, they have helped thousands of people change their lives by reversing insulin resistance and placing diabetes into remission.

How We Can Help You

If you've Googled "how to treat type 2 diabetes," you've probably been bombarded by a lot of conflicting information. Maybe you've read that carbohydrates are bad for diabetes and a low-carb diet is the solution, or that fat is the problem and a low-fat diet is the solution. Unfortunately, these different approaches can be confusing, some of them conflicting, making it challenging to create a clear plan of action. What's more, since type 2 diabetes is a very complex and multifactorial illness (and highly linked to nutrition and lifestyle), it can easily be misunderstood.

While doctors are fully equipped to provide the necessary medications to treat the symptoms of diabetes, they often fail to advise their patients about the available dietary and lifestyle tools that tackle the underlying cause of diabetes: insulin resistance. And no wonder. A study published in the Journal of the Association of American Medical Colleges found that medical students receive less than twenty hours of nutrition education in their four years of medical school, and the average patient visit with a doctor in the United States lasts a mere twenty minutes.

Being told you will have to battle diabetes for the rest of your life can feel overwhelming and frustrating. But what if we told you it didn't have to be this way? We have spent our careers working with a diverse group of people with type 2 diabetes. And we've found that if you're willing to put in the work, you can achieve a life free from diabetes.

Take Sarah as an example. After being diagnosed with type 2 diabetes, she felt helpless. She struggled with an A1c (a measure of blood sugar) of 10.8%, extra weight, high triglycerides, and hair loss. So she did what most people think is the right solution—she stopped eating all carbs and focused on a meat-and-vegetable diet. But after a few months, she still wasn't feeling well, and her diabetes symptoms had worsened. Then she found us and learned about our approach. After two weeks following our guidance, she started seeing results in her blood sugar levels. And after a few months, her doctor was blown away when she returned with her updated bloodwork.

Here's an excerpt from Sarah:

"My doctor could not believe my numbers. My glucose (blood sugar) levels were in the 300s and are now in the 80s and 90s. My doctor said, 'I can't call you a diabetic anymore.' My A1c dropped from 10.8% to 5.5%. On top of that, my triglycerides went from 324 to 65 mg/dL! I've lost 25.3 pounds, my hair has stopped falling out, and the dark circles around my eyes are gone. My whole life changed since starting your program!"

Sarah is just one example of the many people we've had the opportunity of helping. You, too, can achieve results similar to Sarah. But before you dive right into our recipes and meal plan, take a few minutes to read ahead to familiarize yourself with type 2 diabetes and why our approach, when done correctly, works so well to put diabetes into remission and keep it there.

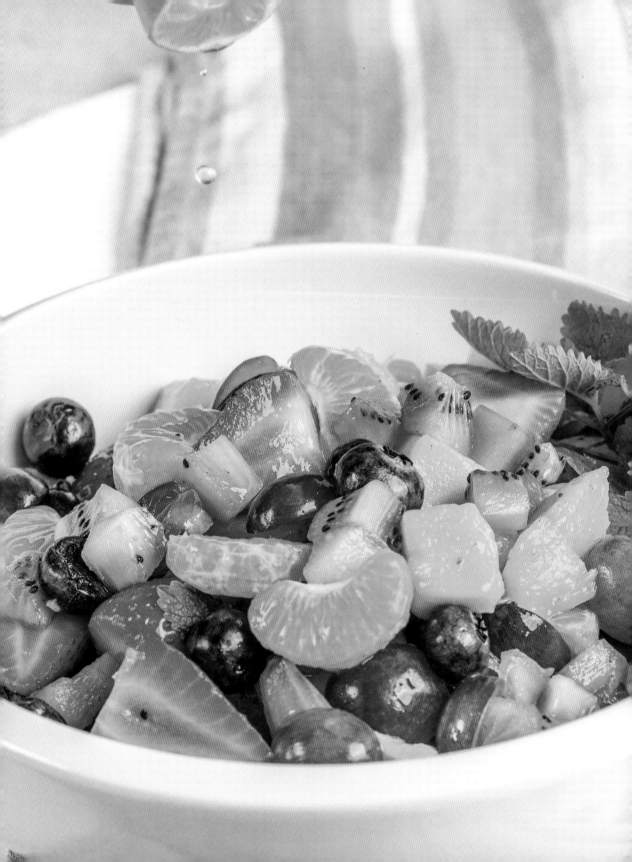

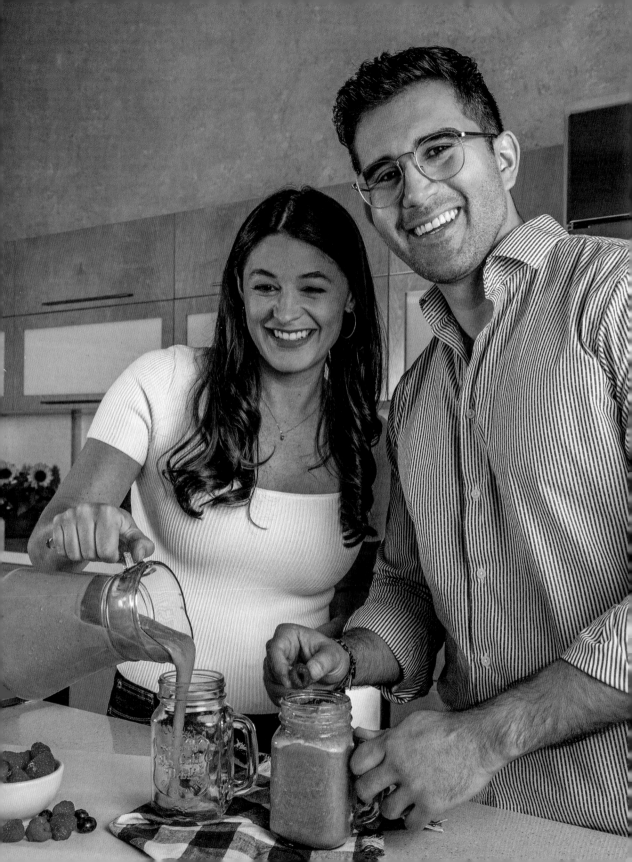

Part 1:
Diet and Nutrition

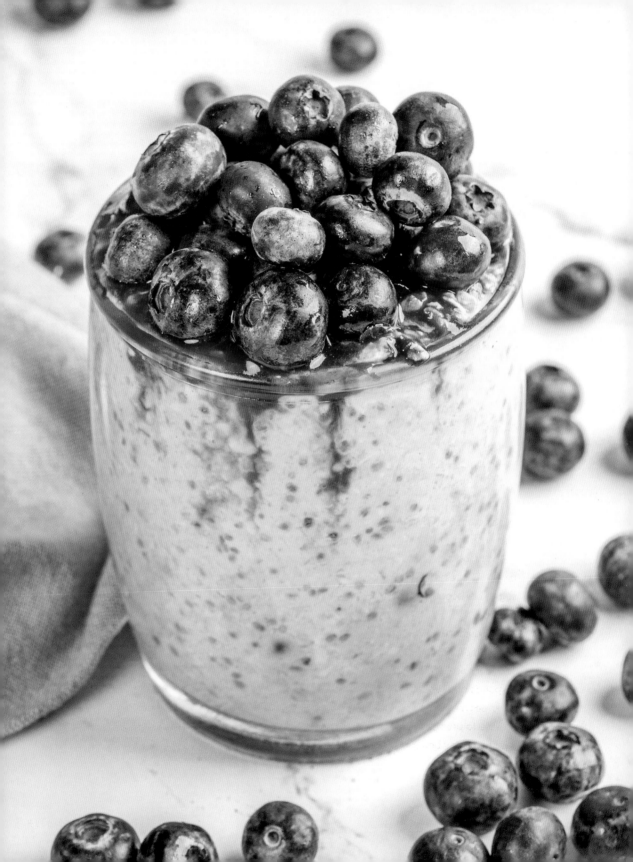

CHAPTER 1

Diabetes Basics

Let's start with the basics. This chapter discusses the foundations of diabetes, how it progresses, and why some people are more prone to developing it than others. We believe that understanding this information is a crucial first step toward putting diabetes into remission. By the end of this chapter, you'll have a deeper understanding of diabetes and feel confident in your knowledge about this condition.

Type 1 vs. Type 2 Diabetes

Diabetes mellitus (DM) is a group of conditions in which the body either does not produce enough, or does not respond normally to, insulin, causing blood glucose (or blood sugar) levels to be abnormally high. Diabetes has many subclassifications, with the main ones being type 1 and type 2.

Type 1 diabetes (T1D) is an autoimmune condition where the body attacks and destroys most of the insulin-producing cells of the pancreas. Insulin keeps blood sugar in check, so without it, blood sugar rises above normal levels. As a result, people with T1D must inject insulin to control their blood sugar. T1D accounts for 5 to 10% of all diabetes cases.

Type 2 diabetes (T2D), on the other hand, is often referred to as *insulin-resistant diabetes* and accounts for 90 to 95% of all diabetes cases. In T2D, cells are unable to properly respond to insulin. The pancreas, in turn, responds by producing even more insulin. If this persists over time, the pancreas may overwork itself, suffer permanent damage, and no longer be able to produce sufficient, or any, insulin at all. At this point, insulin injections may become necessary.

Diagnosis

Diabetes, including prediabetes, can be diagnosed through the several tests outlined below. If diabetes is suspected, a second test must be repeated to confirm the diagnosis.

Diabetes Diagnostic Criteria

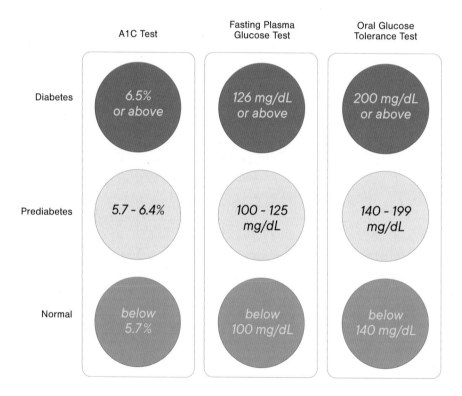

	A1C Test	Fasting Plasma Glucose Test	Oral Glucose Tolerance Test
Diabetes	6.5% or above	126 mg/dL or above	200 mg/dL or above
Prediabetes	5.7 - 6.4%	100 - 125 mg/dL	140 - 199 mg/dL
Normal	below 5.7%	below 100 mg/dL	below 140 mg/dL

A1C

An A1C test, also known as a hemoglobin A1C or HbA1c test, measures your *average* blood glucose over the past two to three months. This test is convenient as it does not require fasting.

Type 2 diabetes is diagnosed at an A1C level of greater than or equal to 6.5%

Fasting Plasma (or Blood) Glucose (FPG)

An FPG test measures your fasting blood glucose levels. It is a simple blood test administered after fasting for at least eight hours, best done in the morning before breakfast.

Type 2 diabetes is diagnosed at a fasting blood glucose level of greater than or equal to 126 mg/dL

Oral Glucose Tolerance Test (OGTT)

An OGTT is a two-hour test that checks your blood glucose levels before and two hours after drinking a special sweet drink. It tells the doctor how your body processes sugar and is the test most commonly used to diagnose gestational diabetes.

Type 2 diabetes is diagnosed at a two-hour blood glucose level of greater than or equal to 200 mg/dL

Random (or Casual) Plasma Glucose Test

A random plasma glucose test is used to check blood glucose levels at any time of the day if severe diabetes symptoms are present.

Type 2 diabetes is diagnosed at a blood glucose level of greater than or equal to 200 mg/dL

How Glucose and Insulin Work in the Body

To understand how type 2 diabetes develops, we need to understand how glucose and insulin function.

Glucose is an essential molecule, and without it, life would not be possible. It's a simple sugar (also known as a monosaccharide, a type of carbohydrate) that our body uses for energy to fuel our brain, muscles, and other organs in our body. But like anything else in our body, glucose must exist in homeostasis—or a state of equilibrium. In other words, to function effectively, glucose must be at the perfect level—not too high, not too low—and insulin is one of the hormones that helps regulate this.

When we eat food that contains carbohydrates (regardless of the kind), the body converts them into glucose. As glucose enters the bloodstream, the pancreas receives a signal to release insulin. As you can see on the following page, insulin acts as a "key," opening up "doors," or glucose channels found on the surface of cells. By opening these channels, insulin allows glucose to funnel out of the bloodstream and into our cells.

How Does Insulin Work?

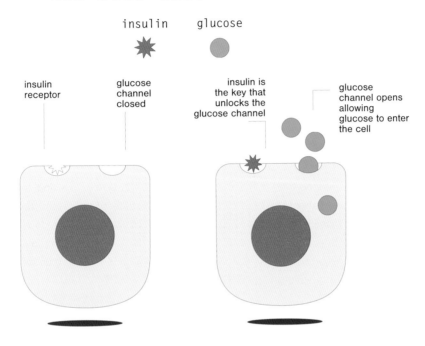

insulin

glucose

insulin receptor

glucose channel closed

insulin is the key that unlocks the glucose channel

glucose channel opens allowing glucose to enter the cell

Once inside our cells, glucose is either immediately used as energy or stored for later use in the form of glycogen. As this process continues, blood glucose levels return to a normal range. This hormonal "check and balance" system keeps blood glucose under control.

In type 2 diabetes, this system becomes impaired, leading to hyperglycemia or high blood glucose. Let's find out why.

How Insulin Resistance Leads to Type 2 Diabetes

Insulin resistance—when cells fail to respond to insulin—is one of the primary causes of type 2 diabetes.

The precise cause of insulin resistance remains unknown, but recent research suggests that a continuous surplus of energy in the body (caused by overeating) plays an important role. Evolutionarily, our bodies were not programmed to waste energy, so any food we consume is either used right away or stored as fat for later use. Unfortunately, our bodies contain a finite number of adipose (fat) cells, and there is a limit to how much fat they can hold. When these cells reach their capacity, they swell up and produce an inflammatory response. This response obstructs insulin's role as a "key," ultimately leaving fewer doors open and more glucose trapped in the blood.

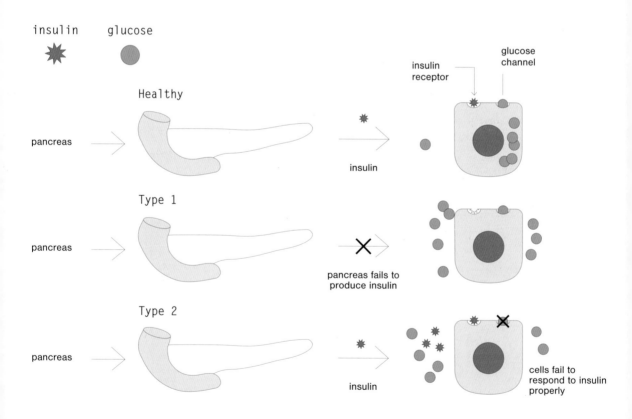

insulin

glucose

insulin receptor

glucose channel

Healthy

pancreas

insulin

Type 1

pancreas

pancreas fails to produce insulin

Type 2

pancreas

insulin

cells fail to respond to insulin properly

Researchers are also studying saturated fat's role in the development of insulin resistance. Research suggests that replacing saturated fat with unsaturated sources significantly improves insulin sensitivity (more on this in Chapter 2).

Regardless, over the course of time, if nothing is done to stop and reverse insulin resistance, blood glucose levels will continue to rise, eventually reaching the classification of prediabetes and, ultimately, type 2 diabetes. Currently, 96 million Americans (more than one in three) have prediabetes, yet more than 80% don't know they have it. Prediabetes is a silent disease. It doesn't show many signs or symptoms and can easily go undetected for months or even years. If left untreated, many people with prediabetes will go on to develop type 2 diabetes, which currently affects 33 to 35 million Americans.

The good news is that you can prevent prediabetes from turning into type 2 diabetes through weight loss and physical activity. The landmark 2002 Diabetes Prevention Program trial showed that when people achieved a 7% reduction in body weight and engaged in at least 150 minutes of physical activity per week, they reduced their incidence of type 2 diabetes by 58%!

However, without any lifestyle changes, diabetes worsens. As the pancreas senses that blood sugar is still high, it secretes even more insulin (more "keys") in hopes of opening more cell "doors" to bring blood sugar down to normal. As this process continues, the pancreas becomes overworked, which leads to the death of its beta cells (the cells responsible for making insulin). As a result, natural insulin production decreases, and it becomes necessary to supply the body with insulin via injection.

What Increases Your Risk of Prediabetes and Type 2 Diabetes?

Type 2 diabetes is a multifactorial condition, meaning many factors may play a role in its development. However, excess body fat, especially around the abdominal area, is one of the strongest risk factors for type 2 diabetes, and almost always causes some degree of insulin resistance. Other common risk factors for type 2 diabetes include the following:

- Having prediabetes
- Being 45 years of age or older
- Having an immediate family member with type 2 diabetes
- Having a history of gestational diabetes
- Being a certain race and ethnicity, such as African American, Hispanic or Latino, Pacific Islander, American Indian, or Alaska Native

While type 2 diabetes appears to be related to family history in immediate family members (i.e., a parent or sibling), the genetics of type 2 diabetes are still poorly understood. As Dr. Caldwell Esselstyn's popular analogy goes, "genetics loads the gun, lifestyle pulls the trigger." Even if you have a family history of type 2 diabetes, you still have the power to prevent its onset with your lifestyle choices. Of course, genes aren't the only thing we inherit from our parents. Children often adopt their family's eating habits and exercise patterns, making it difficult to determine which contributes more to the inheritability of type 2 diabetes: genes or passed-down behaviors.

Long-Term Complications of Type 2 Diabetes

If left untreated over a long period of time, type 2 diabetes may lead to long-term health complications, which include heart disease, chronic kidney disease, and nerve damage. This section isn't meant to frighten or intimidate you, but rather to make you aware of the very real and life-threatening long-term complications of type 2 diabetes. Fortunately, by changing your diet and lifestyle, you can significantly reduce your risk of these events.

Heart Disease

Over time, high amounts of sugar in the blood can damage the delicate blood vessels and nerves of the heart. People with diabetes are twice as likely to have a heart attack or stroke than someone without diabetes. Heart disease is the leading cause of death for people with diabetes, and sadly, more than 65% of people with type 2 diabetes die from cardiovascular complications, such as heart attacks, strokes, and heart failure.

Kidney Disease

Diabetes can also damage blood vessels in the kidneys. As this damage accumulates, the kidneys' ability to function declines. Over 30% of people with diabetes will also have kidney disease. In fact, diabetes is the leading cause of kidney disease in the United States.

Nerve Damage

Persistently high blood sugar levels can also damage nerves (important tissues that send signals between the brain and parts of your body). Diabetes-related nerve damage (diabetic peripheral neuropathy), which affects nearly half of all diabetes sufferers, causes pain and numbness in the extremities. And more than 30% of people with diabetes have autonomic neuropathy, nerve damage related to the internal organs. You may not notice any symptoms related to nerve damage until that damage becomes severe.

Foot Problems

Diabetes may restrict the amount of blood flow to the feet, making it difficult for ulcers, sores, and infections to heal; in extreme cases, this can lead to amputations. Not surprisingly, diabetes is one of the leading causes of amputations in the United States. It is vital to check your feet regularly and to maintain proper foot hygiene.

Vision Loss

Diabetic retinopathy (eye damage due to diabetes) is the top cause of blindness in working-age adults. High blood glucose causes the blood vessels in the retina (the light-sensitive layer of cells in the back of the eye) to swell and leak, leading to blurred vision.

Can Type 2 Diabetes Be Reversed or Put Into Remission?

Most research published to date shows that many individuals with type 2 diabetes can reach normal glucose levels after adopting dietary interventions that lead to weight loss. The Counterpoint, Counterbalance, and DiRECT trials are among the major studies that show how low-calorie diets, accompanied by weight loss, can put diabetes into remission.

While a very low-calorie diet can lead to diabetes remission, this approach is challenging, especially without a structured program and medical supervision. So, what is the best and safest way to reverse type 2 diabetes?

The American Diabetes Association (ADA) says that a variety of eating plans can safely and efficiently help people with diabetes achieve weight loss. They cite the Mediterranean-style, low-carbohydrate, and vegetarian or plant-based eating patterns as examples of healthful diets that have shown positive results for individuals with type 2 diabetes.

Keeping type 2 diabetes in remission depends on sustained weight loss. The more restrictive a diet, the less likely it is to be followed in the long-term, leading to weight regain and the return of type 2 diabetes.

So, what is the dietary pattern we recommend—regardless of whether you need to lose weight or not—that has helped thousands of our clients put diabetes in remission and keep it there? We'll review this in Chapter 2.

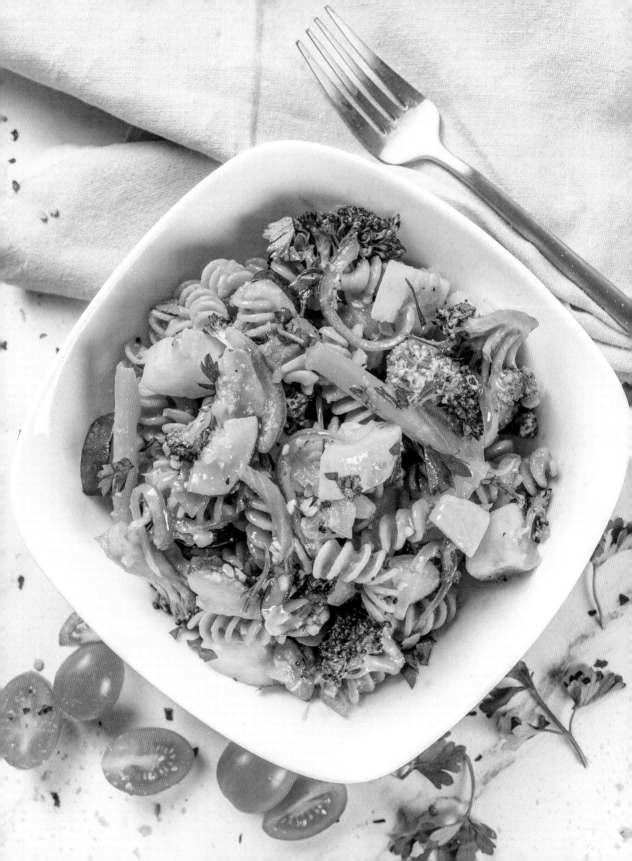

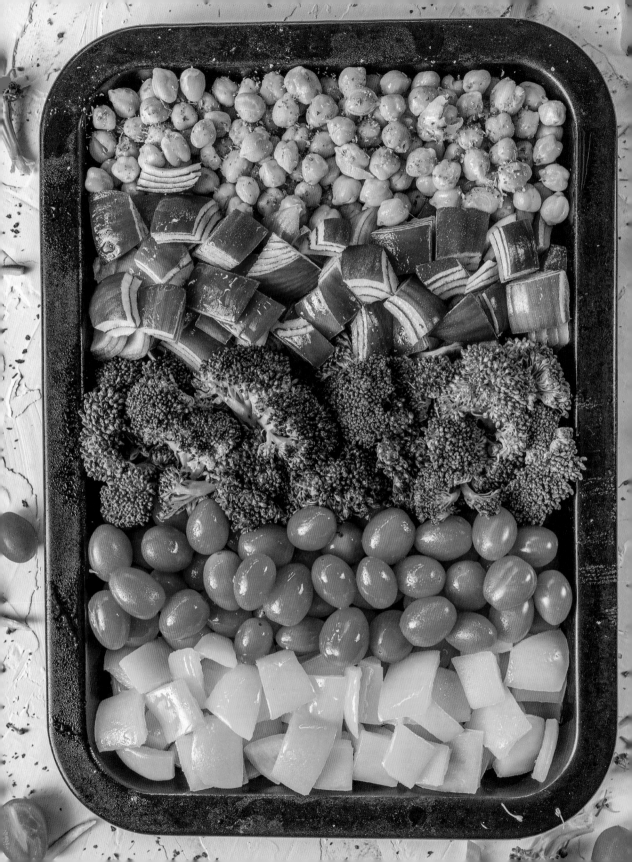

CHAPTER 2

Placing Diabetes into Remission with a (Mostly) Plant-Based Diet

The word "diet" is often associated with a person making a drastic change to their food choices to lose weight, inevitably involving food restriction, deprivation, or calorie counting. Such "diets" may result in some weight loss, but are often hard to sustain, leading to weight regain, followed by a new diet—a cycle referred to as yo-yo dieting.

Our approach is devoid of fads and trends, stops and starts. It presents a dietary framework that will support good health for the rest of your life. It focuses on an "80/20 dietary pattern" where 80% of your diet comes from nutrient-dense foods, while the remaining 20% offers flexibility for more calorie-dense options. Let's discuss why we recommend this approach and the difference between calorie-dense vs. nutrient-dense foods.

Nutrient Density vs. Calorie Density

Americans are consuming excess calories from less nutritious foods thanks to the accessibility and palatability of ultra-processed foods and animal-based foods. Ultra-processed foods have many added ingredients such as sugar, salt, fat, and artificial colors or preservatives, and are calorie-dense, meaning they're high in calories with few nutrients. Examples of ultra-processed foods include breakfast cereals, chips, ice cream, processed meats like hot dogs and deli meats, sugary drinks, and bakery products like muffins and cakes. Animal-based foods have also become extremely accessible. While they are a rich source of protein, animal-based foods also contain higher amounts of saturated fat and no fiber. Eating these foods frequently can lead to overconsumption of calories, which can lead to excess weight—a contributor of insulin resistance.

Nutrient-dense foods, on the other hand, are rich in nutrients such as vitamins, minerals, and antioxidants, and low in calories, since they contain little to no added sugar or saturated fat. And because nutrient-dense foods tend to be lower in calories, you can eat a lot more of them, which helps fill you up and keep you full for longer.

Calorie Density vs. Nutrient Density

800 calories

Low volume

Low nutrient density

Low satiety (unsatisfied)

800 calories

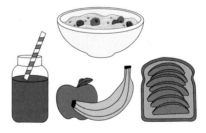

High(er) volume

High(er) nutrient density

More satiating (satisfied)

Most nutrient-dense foods fall into five major categories: fruits, vegetables, legumes (beans, lentils, and peas), whole grains, and nuts and seeds. If 80% of your diet comes from these plant-based, whole foods, then you will be establishing a solid foundation for optimal health and longevity.

Did you know the people who live the longest have eating habits similar to the 80/20 pattern? In 2004, explorer Dan Buettner teamed up with National Geographic and the National Institute of Aging to lead an expedition around the world to unearth the secrets of longevity. Using epidemiological data, statistics, birth certificates, and other research, Buettner discovered five locations, called the "Blue Zones," with the highest percentage of centenarians—people who live to be at least 100 years old. Perhaps even more interesting, the majority of these people not only reached 100, but they also lived with virtually no chronic illnesses like diabetes, heart disease, obesity, cancer, or dementia. Buettner discovered that a common characteristic among the people in these five locations was their diet, which included whole, unrefined foods, very little meat, and daily consumption of fruits, vegetables, whole grains, and legumes!

Dan Buettner's findings weren't far off from what the total body of evidence shows. Plant-based or plant-predominant diets not only improve longevity but can reduce the risk of type 2 diabetes, treat type 2 diabetes, and reduce key diabetes-related complications. As additional corroborating research emerges, more organizations are recognizing and supporting this way of eating.

The American Diabetes Association's 2023 Standards of Care recognized a plant-based dietary pattern as an effective way to treat type 2 diabetes. The American Heart Association stated in their 2021 Dietary Guidance to Improve Cardiovascular Health that the majority of our proteins should be plant-based (remember, people with type 2 diabetes face a greater risk of heart disease). In their 2020 guidelines, the American Association of Clinical Endocrinology encouraged their clinicians to recommend a primarily plant-based diet rich in healthful carbohydrates and low in saturated fat to their patients with type 2 diabetes. And in 2021, the American College of Lifestyle Medicine came to a consensus that for long-term remission of type 2 diabetes, individuals should focus on changing their style of diet, adopting a style such as a Mediterranean, DASH, or whole-food, plant-based diet, instead of simply focusing on specific nutrients (e.g., low-carbohydrate, low-fat, high-protein).

The Elements of a Plant-Based Diet for Type 2 Diabetes

Why does a plant-based, whole-food diet work so well to not only help you live longer but also reduce your risk of diabetes and other chronic diseases? Let's review a few of the key components.

Nutrient-Dense: High in Fiber and Antioxidants

Plant-based diets are high in fiber and antioxidants, both of which have been shown to improve glycemic control and insulin sensitivity. Fiber, a type of carbohydrate only found in plant-based foods, cannot be digested or absorbed. Because of this, it slows down the absorption of sugar from food, thereby minimizing spikes in blood sugar after eating. Research shows that fiber intake improves HbA1c, fasting blood sugar, fasting insulin, and insulin resistance. Fiber also promotes satiety and has been linked with weight loss, which in turn lowers insulin resistance. As fiber travels down our intestinal tract and reaches our large intestine, it serves as food for our gut bacteria. As the bacteria gobble it up in a process called fermentation, they release a byproduct called short-chain fatty acids (or SCFAs). These SCFAs have been shown to improve glucose response, insulin signaling, insulin sensitivity, and pancreatic dysfunction. Lastly, fiber has been associated with reducing markers of inflammation, which may also improve insulin resistance.

Unfortunately, only 7% of Americans meet the daily fiber recommendations of 25 grams a day for women and 38 grams a day for men. Fiber is found in all plant-based foods, so eating a (mostly) plant-based diet can ensure you reach your fiber requirement.

Dietary antioxidants are substances found in food that help to protect cells from damage. Foods rich in antioxidants have been shown to decrease the absorption of glucose into the bloodstream, stimulate insulin secretion, and improve the uptake of glucose into cells. Plant-based foods, especially fruits and vegetables, are rich sources of antioxidants. Like fiber, antioxidants are best consumed from whole-food sources. Antioxidant supplements have not been shown to prevent disease.

Low in Saturated Fat

There are two main types of dietary fat: unsaturated and saturated. Saturated fat has been linked to insulin resistance and an increased risk of type 2 diabetes due to a phenomenon known as lipotoxicity. Excess saturated fat intake accumulates in the cells of the liver and muscles—two organs not designed to store fat. Lipotoxicity impairs insulin signaling, as you may remember from Chapter 1, insulin is responsible for opening the cell's "doors" or glucose channels. As lipotoxicity develops, less glucose is funneled into cells and more remains trapped in the blood. Conversely, unsaturated fat can improve glycemic control, especially when it replaces saturated fat in the diet. Saturated fat is found primarily in animal-based foods (as well as in coconut and palm); therefore, a more plant-based diet will be naturally lower in saturated fat.

Promotes a Healthy Body Weight

Lastly, a plant-based diet promotes weight and fat loss, which is important because excess weight and fat are two major contributors to insulin resistance. On the other hand, meat, refined grains, and added sugars have all been implicated in weight gain and insulin resistance. The availability and tastiness of these foods make them easier to overconsume, which may lead to weight gain. A whole-foods, plant-based dietary approach not only excludes animal products, but also minimizes the intake of refined grains and added sugars. On both accounts, plant-based foods can help you shed excess weight and boost your insulin sensitivity.

Improving Your Tolerance to Carbohydrates

We know what you may be thinking right now: "But some of these plant-based foods spike my glucose levels!" Yes, they may, but that's not because these foods are bad for you; it's because your cells can't adequately respond to insulin. A rise in blood sugar after a meal is normal. However, an *abnormally* high rise in blood sugar indicates insulin resistance.

Blood Glucose Levels after a Meal

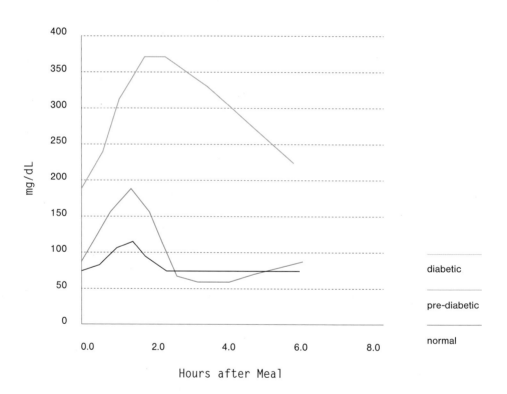

But simply avoiding all carbohydrates is not a solution. By following a nutrient-dense, whole-foods, plant-based eating pattern, you will ideally be able to regain your insulin sensitivity and improve your body's tolerance to carbohydrates over time. This is how you'll be able to tell that you're well on your way to placing your diabetes into remission. If you don't typically check your blood sugar after meals, then use your fasting blood glucose to monitor your insulin sensitivity. Read about what our program member Charlie had to say about his ability to tolerate carbs again:

> *"I can't tell you the value of being able to eat fruit again. I'm now able to enjoy bananas and peaches again! It's such a delight! My medication has been cut in half, my insulin has been cut in half, and I've dropped about 13 pounds since the start of the program. The program truly opened my eyes to plant-based eating. I love the program, and I've recommended it to multiple people."*

As always, if you are taking glucose-lowering medications, consult with your physician before changing your diet.

Vegan vs. Whole-Food Plant-Based Eating

We want to emphasize that we are not recommending a strict vegan or vegetarian diet, but rather a nutrient-dense, whole-foods one that is predominantly plant-based (about 80%) while allowing for the consumption of animal products and more processed foods (20%). Many people find vegan and vegetarian diets too restrictive or too inflexible. We understand this—hence the 20% allowance for other foods, should you choose to add them. Remember, vegan doesn't always mean healthier, either, as a vegan diet still allows foods such as fried potato chips, OREO cookies, fake meats, and highly sweetened soft drinks.

Given that we're not recommending a strictly vegan diet, you may wonder why all our meal plans and recipes are fully plant-based. There are two reasons:

1) Most people already know how to include meat and dairy in their meals, but fewer are able to prepare delicious, satiating plant-based meals that they'll look forward to eating. The variety, tastes, textures, and flavor profiles of a plant-based dietary approach are boundless, and we're excited to help you find the joy in plant-based cooking and eating.

2) We believe adopting a fully plant-based diet is the quickest way to reverse insulin resistance, regain control of your blood sugar levels, and minimize your risk of diabetes complications. For this reason, we suggest beginning with a four-week meal plan that is completely plant-based. At the end of the four weeks, if you'd like to re-introduce animal products, we'll show you the best way to do so in Chapter 6: Beyond the Four Weeks (page 93). If you prefer not to, or cannot, do the meal plan completely plant-based, then focus on lean animal-based foods such as fish and shellfish, egg whites, and low-fat yogurt. But the more you stick to a 100% plant-based diet, the more likely you are to see greater results.

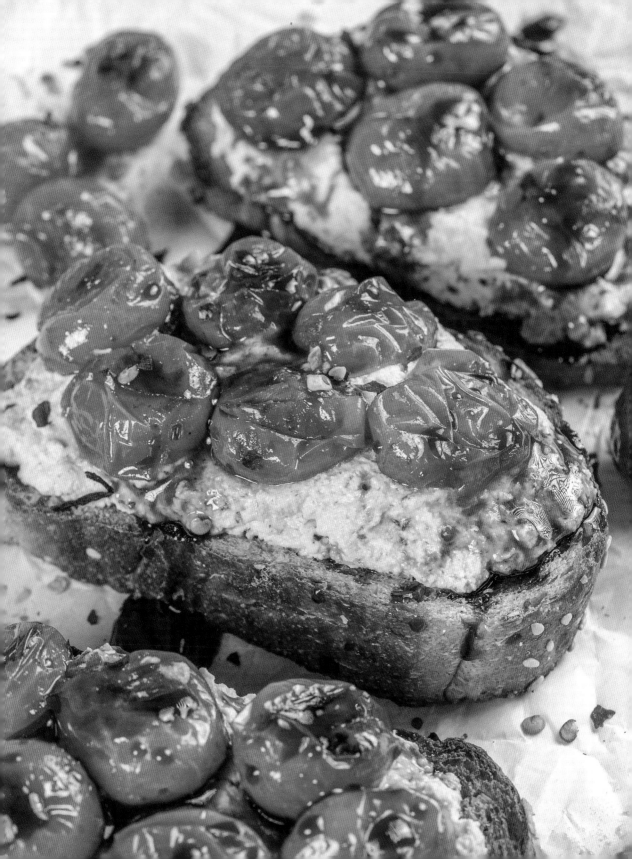

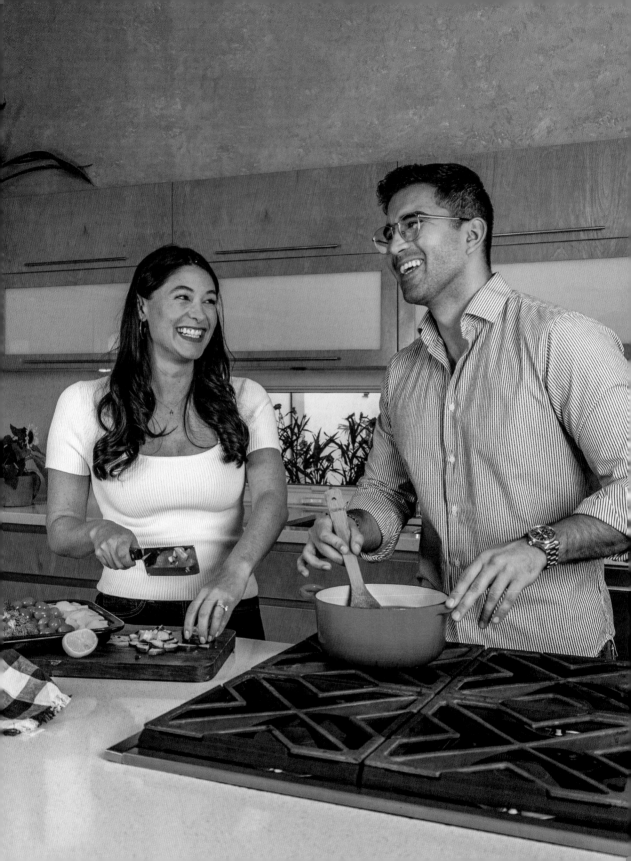

Part 2:
The Meal Plan

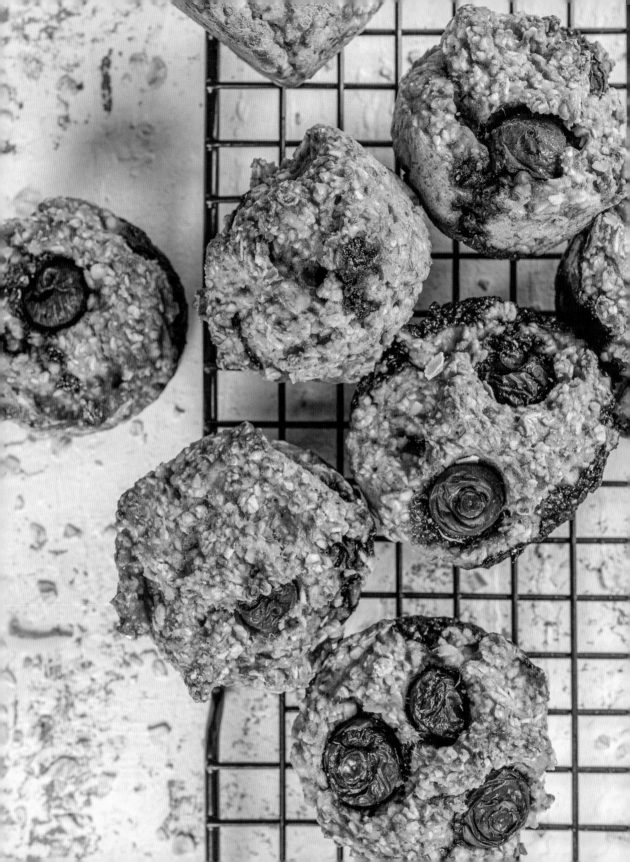

CHAPTER 3

Preparing for the Meal Plan and Recipes

To reiterate, our meal plan is 100% plant-based because we believe it is the quickest way to reverse insulin resistance, regain control of your blood sugar levels, and prevent long-term diabetes complications. Soon, you'll be able to enjoy high-fiber carbohydrates without experiencing abnormally high blood sugar spikes. Don't feel that you need to rush into the meal plan. It's always best to start by making dietary changes that you're comfortable with. If you feel intimidated or overwhelmed when starting a meal plan, remember you will still benefit simply by incorporating more plant-based meals into your diet.

If you're ready to dive into this meal plan and try a plant-based diet for four weeks, then we're excited to help get you started. Take a moment to read these next two chapters, which tell you everything you need to know to succeed. Each week of the meal plan includes a grocery list, snack and dessert options, and guidance on how to best prep your meals for the week ahead.

While we would love to accommodate everyone's dietary preferences, it's impossible for us to do so. We do our best to provide gluten-free options and ingredient swap suggestions for the top allergens in the United States (which include tree nuts, peanuts, wheat, and soy) when possible. Many ingredients are easily interchangeable, so feel free to get creative with the foods you prefer.

How Does It Work?

Each week's meal plan includes a complete shopping list, a weekend meal-prep to-do list, and a full weekly menu of breakfasts, lunches, and dinners, which you can make using the recipes in this book. We also provide suggestions for snacks and desserts. The meal plan is structured assuming you will shop and do some meal prep over the weekend, but it can be adjusted to suit your lifestyle. If a specific meal doesn't appeal to you, feel free to swap it for another one. All meals are completely interchangeable.

Unlimited Non-Starchy Veggies

Yes, you read that correctly: on this plan, there is no limit to the number of non-starchy veggies you can eat! Non-starchy vegetables are a perfect example of nutrient-dense foods; they are low in carbohydrates and calories but packed with vitamins, minerals, and fiber. They are the ideal food to help fill you up while keeping your blood sugar in check. In fact, the more of these foods you can include in your daily meals, the better it will be for your overall health. So if you want more spinach in a meal or baby carrots in your snack, go for it!

Here's a list of common non-starchy vegetables:

- Artichokes
- Asparagus
- Baby corn
- Bamboo shoots
- Bean sprouts
- Beets
- Brussels sprouts
- Broccoli
- Cabbage (green, bok choy, Chinese)
- Carrots
- Cauliflower
- Celery
- Chayote
- Cucumber
- Daikon
- Eggplant
- Green beans (string beans, Italian/runner beans, wax beans)
- Greens (collard, kale, mustard, turnip)
- Hearts of palm
- Jicama
- Kohlrabi
- Leeks
- Mushrooms
- Okra
- Onions
- Peppers
- Radishes
- Rutabagas
- Salad greens (chicory, endive, escarole, lettuce, romaine, spinach, arugula, radicchio, watercress)
- Sprouts
- Squash (cushaw, summer, crookneck, spaghetti, zucchini)
- Sugar snap peas
- Swiss chard
- Tomatoes
- Turnips
- Water chestnuts
- Yardlong beans

Recipe Nutritional Information

With every recipe, we've listed the Calories, Fat, Carbs, Fiber, Protein, and Carb-to-Fiber Ratio. This nutritional information was calculated for every recipe exactly as written, without any extra toppings or swaps, including optional ingredients. Of course, the information may change based on what products you use—for example, one non-dairy milk may have more protein and less fat than another—but the nutritional information listed here will serve as a basic guideline. We tested our recipes with Silk's Unsweetened Soymilk, Kite Hill's Unsweetened Plain Almondmilk Yogurt, Sunwarrior's Vanilla Protein Powder, Kirkland's Creamy Peanut Butter, and Lily's Dark Chocolate Baking Chips.

Carb-to-Fiber Ratio

As you may remember from Chapter 2, fiber is a type of carbohydrate that is not digested or absorbed by the body and slows the absorption of sugar into the bloodstream. Therefore, the more fiber in the carbohydrates you eat, the better control you'll have over your blood sugar. A report from the Harvard School of Public Health recommends using the 10:1 ratio rule for choosing grain products, which states that for every 10 grams of carbohydrate, there should be at least 1 gram of fiber. We applied this principle to our recipes and kept most of our recipes below a ratio of 6:1. You can easily figure out the carb-to-fiber ratio of any food by simply dividing the carbohydrates by the fiber, in the nutrition information provided here. In most cases, we rounded to the nearest integer, unless shown otherwise. So you can rest assured that even though you're eating more carbohydrates with this dietary pattern, you're also consuming plenty of fiber.

Increasing Calories on the Meal Plan

Your recommended calorie intake for the day depends on various factors, such as your age, sex, height, weight, and activity level. But generally, most women need 1,600 to 2,400 calories per day to maintain their weight, while most men need 2,000 to 3,000 calories. Eating less than your recommended calorie intake leads to weight loss.

We can't match the calorie requirements for everyone in a single meal plan, so let your hunger and satiety signals guide you on this journey. If a meal doesn't quite fill you up, then that's a sign you may need another serving of it. Or if you find that you're hungry between meals, have a snack! The meal plans in Chapter 5 only include breakfast, lunch, and dinner, but you should feel free to incorporate snacks and desserts as you see fit. You can choose from the nutritionally balanced snack and dessert recipes in this book, or take advantage of the unlimited non-starchy veggies allowed on this meal plan, for any between-meal snacking. You shouldn't feel hungry on this meal plan. If you do, it's a sign that you're not eating enough.

Tips for Success

Mindset and Motivation

Mindset matters when starting a new dietary plan. Understanding your "why" is a powerful motivator. Before you begin, grab a piece of paper and write down the reasons why you are embarking on this meal plan and dietary program.

A "why" statement can look like this:

"I want to lose 15 pounds and drop my A1c by 1 to 2% within the next three to four months so I can reduce my need for medications, prevent diabetes complications, and extend my quality of life. I want to see my children and grandchildren grow up and I want to be able to spend family time without having to worry about any health issues."

Once you have written down your "why," post it where you will see it several times a day, such as on your bathroom mirror, behind your house door, or on your fridge. This will serve as motivation and will help remind you why you've started this journey, especially when times get tough.

Meal Prep

Preparing and cooking meals at home saves time, money, and calories—standard restaurant meals tend to have more calories, fat, refined carbohydrates, and sodium than home-cooked meals—but for many of us it's hard to find the time to cook at home every day. Meal prepping not only makes weekday cooking easier, it can also directly improve your diabetes health. A study found that after completing a meal-prep program, participants with type 2 diabetes experienced improvements in eating control, body weight, HbA1c levels, and blood pressure. Meal prepping works, and it will be essential in helping you succeed with the meal plan. Each week, we provide tips on what to meal prep over the weekend to save you time in the kitchen during the week.

Stocking Your Kitchen with Essentials

Stocking your fridge, freezer, and pantry with healthy, diabetes-friendly ingredients will make meal preparation and cooking much easier. Below, we've listed a few of the pantry, fridge, and freezer staples that will help you throughout the meal plan. We've also listed our favorite kitchen tools and appliances, which you'll need to prepare many of the recipes in this book.

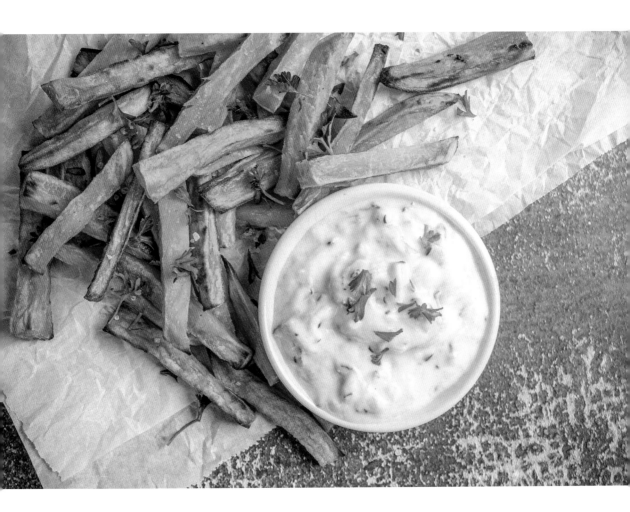

To Keep in Your Pantry:

Beans and Other Canned/Bottled Goods:

- Black beans (canned and/or dry)
- Bottled lemon/lime juice
- Chickpeas (canned and/or dry)
- Light coconut milk
- Diced tomatoes
- Kidney beans (canned and/or dry)
- Lentils (canned and/or dry)
- Pasta sauce
- Pinto beans (canned and/or dry)
- Salsa
- Tomato paste
- Tomato sauce
- White beans (canned and/or dry)

Whole Grains and Pastas:

- Brown rice
- Brown rice noodles
- Chickpea pasta
- Farro
- Lentil pasta
- Millet
- Oats (steel-cut and rolled)
- Quinoa
- Whole-wheat pasta

Nuts and Seeds:

- Almonds
- Brazil nuts
- Cashews
- Chia seeds
- Ground flaxseed (also called flax meal)
- Hemp seeds (also called hemp hearts)
- Peanut, almond, or sunflower seed butter
- Pine nuts
- Pumpkin seeds
- Sunflower seeds
- Tahini
- Walnuts

Dried Herbs and Spices:

- Bay leaves
- Cayenne
- Chili powder
- Curry powder
- Dried oregano
- Dried mint
- Ginger
- Ground cinnamon
- Ground cumin
- Garam masala
- Garlic powder
- Ground turmeric
- Onion powder
- Paprika
- Red pepper flakes
- Salt and pepper

Vinegars and Condiments:

- Apple cider vinegar
- Balsamic vinegar
- Mustard (yellow and Dijon)
- Olive oil cooking spray
- Rice vinegar
- Tamari, less-sodium soy sauce, or coconut aminos

Other:

- Cocoa powder
- Dates
- Monk fruit sweetener
- No-sugar-added chocolate chips
- Nutritional yeast
- Popcorn kernels
- Protein powder
- Rice paper sheets
- Shelf-stable non-dairy milk
- Vanilla extract
- Vegetable broth

To Keep in Your Fridge:

- Fresh fruit
- Fresh vegetables
- Hummus
- Non-dairy yogurt
- Pesto
- Salad dressings
- Tempeh
- Tofu
- Vegan mayonnaise

To Keep in Your Freezer:

- Banana (peel and freeze ripe bananas)
- Berries
- Cauliflower rice
- Edamame
- Peas
- Spinach and/or kale
- Stir-fry veggies
- Strawberries
- Veggie burgers

Helpful Kitchen Tools and Appliances:

- High-powered blender: great for blending larger batches of food like sauces, smoothies, ice cream, and sorbets
- Food processor: helps with food prep by chopping, mincing, mixing, and blending
- Instant Pot®, or other electric multi-cooker: allows you to quickly make grains, beans, and other foods
- Air fryer: great way to "fry" foods without the need for oil
- Tofu press: not essential, but helpful in removing excess liquid from tofu; see "How to Press Tofu" on page 49
- Food storage containers: preferably glass, not plastic; great for leftovers and meal prepping
- Mason jars: use different sizes for overnight oats, salads, soups, smoothies, and other foods on the go
- Veggie chopper: not essential, but helps save time chopping vegetables
- Reusable zipper-lock bags: saves money on traditional plastic storage bags; great for taking snacks on the go
- Measuring spoons and cups
- Spiralizer: great for making noodles out of vegetables (zucchini noodles, sweet potato noodles, etc.)
- Good chef's knives
- Silicone baking mat: helps with oil-free baking

Working with Tofu

As you'll read in Chapter 4: Frequently Asked Questions about the Meal Plan (page 51), soy makes an excellent replacement for meat and provides an abundance of health benefits. We offer various ways to include tofu, which is made from soy, in your diet, including in soups, tacos, sauces, and more. So if you find that tofu isn't your favorite in one recipe, don't let that stop you from trying another.

People often shy away from tofu because they don't know how to cook it, but don't give up on this healthy food. Preparation is key. Water is added to tofu during the packaging process to prevent it from drying out. Extracting that water before cooking prevents it from being soggy and allows it to absorb flavors.

For best results, follow the steps below to press tofu before using it in a recipe.

1) Wrap tofu in a layer of paper towels or a clean dishcloth.

2) Place a weight, such as a book or a large can of food, on the tofu to squeeze out the water.

3) Let the tofu sit for at least thirty minutes. The weight will gradually and effectively squeeze the moisture out of the block of tofu, where it will be absorbed by the paper towels or dishcloth.

4) If the paper towels or dishcloth become fully saturated, you may need to replace them with fresh ones and continue pressing until they are no longer absorbing moisture.

How to Press Tofu

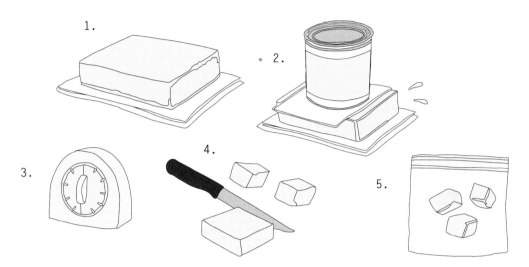

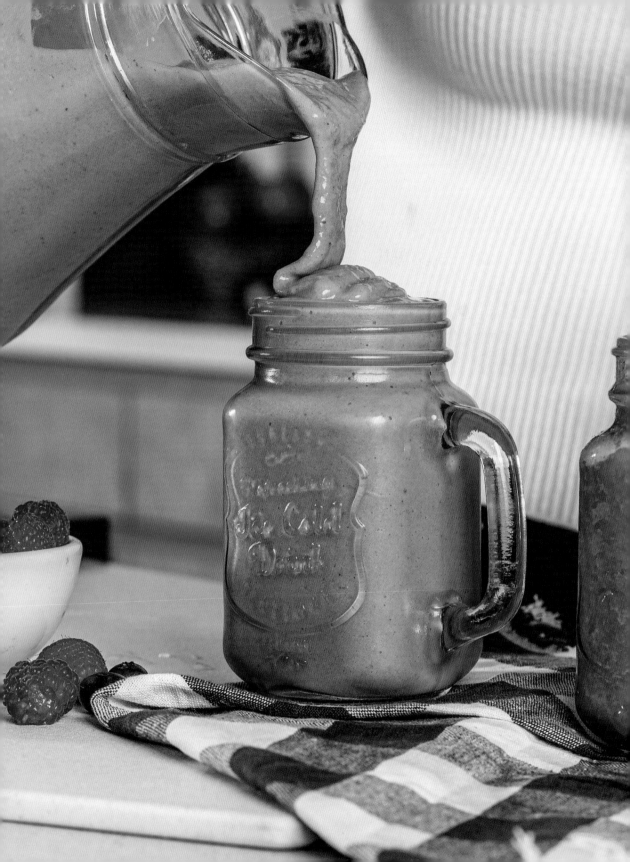

CHAPTER 4

Frequently Asked Questions about the Meal Plan

In this chapter, we've addressed the most frequent questions our clients ask us when starting a plant-based meal plan for diabetes.

What Can I Drink During the Meal Plan?

Water and Sugar-Free Drinks

Maintaining proper hydration is key as you consume more fiber-rich, plant-based foods. Fiber requires water to be digested, so drinking sufficient water will help you maintain regular bowel movements and keep you bloat-free. On average, we should drink nine to thirteen cups (1 cup = 8 ounces) of water daily. Those who are physically active or live in warm climates may need more. If you have trouble reaching these levels, try herbal teas, sparkling flavored waters (with no sugar added), or water infused with herbs and fruit. Staying properly hydrated can also help us feel satiated. Many times we confuse thirst for hunger. Next time you feel hungry, before grabbing a snack, try having a big glass of water, then wait a few minutes and see how you feel.

Coffee and Tea

Coffee and teas are allowed and encouraged on this meal plan! Some individuals notice a small rise in blood sugar after consuming coffee (even black coffee), but the overall body of evidence indicates that coffee can reduce your risk of type 2 diabetes. However, if you're not a coffee drinker or prefer to avoid it, there is no need to start drinking it now. If you do enjoy coffee and/or tea, focus on the ingredients you add to your cup. We recommend using unsweetened non-dairy milk or creamer and avoiding added sugar. Dairy creamers such as half-and-half tend to be rich in saturated fat. Check out the Appendix (page 248) to see our favorite non-dairy creamers.

Non-Dairy Milk

Non-dairy milk is a delicious alternative to regular dairy milk. You'll see that we call for "non-dairy milk" in a handful of our recipes. We generally prefer soy milk over other varieties as it's protein-rich and provides a creamy consistency in recipes. Therefore, we used soy milk in our calculations for the nutrition information for recipes containing milk. However, feel free to use your favorite non-dairy milk, such as almond, oat, coconut, or any other non-dairy variety. Most non-dairy milks can be used interchangeably in these recipes, but we recommend always buying the unsweetened version.

Drinks to Avoid

We encourage you to remove all sugar-sweetened beverages (SSB) from your diet as you embark on this journey. SSB include drinks such as non-diet soft drinks/sodas, flavored juice drinks, sports drinks, sweetened tea and coffee drinks, and energy drinks. If you are accustomed to drinking these beverages, try switching to their diet alternatives, which can save you large amounts of calories and added sugar. For example, a can of Coca-Cola has 39 grams, or 10 teaspoons, of added sugar, while a can of Diet Coke has 0 grams of added sugar. We also recommend avoiding juice and store-bought smoothies, as they tend to contain little to no fiber. For a healthier alternative, try one of our smoothie recipes on page 116.

What Sweeteners May I Use on the Meal Plan?

Dates and Other Fruit

Ideally, the sweetness in your meals should come from foods that have naturally-occuring sugars, not from added sugars. Added sugars are not naturally found in foods; instead, they are added during processing. Check the ingredients list of most store-bought products and you may find added sugar under the guise of dextrose, brown rice syrup, high fructose corn syrup, and many other names. Even natural sweeteners like honey, agave nectar, maple syrup, coconut sugar, and molasses are still considered sources of added sugar, even though they are less processed and may have some nutritional value.

The American Heart Association (AHA) recommends limiting added sugar to 6 teaspoons (or 24 grams) a day for women and 9 teaspoons (or 36 grams) for men. Minimizing added sugars is important for several reasons. For starters, they are a source of "empty calories" that provide little to no nutritional value. Added sugar either displaces more nutrient-dense sources of calories or contributes to an increase in overall calorie intake, which can lead to weight gain. In addition, both added sugars and refined grains elevate blood sugar levels more than fruits, vegetables, and whole grains, all of which contain fiber.

We avoid added sugar in our recipes, and instead turn to naturally sweet ingredients such as fruit, dates, and monk fruit to satisfy a sweet tooth. Given the innumerable health benefits of consuming fruit, we prefer to sweeten recipes with whole fruits when possible. You may notice dates in a few of our recipes. Dates are a naturally sweet fruit packed with lots of nutrients, and contain antioxidants, fiber, and micronutrients like potassium and vitamin B6. We chose dates as a sweetener in many of our dessert recipes so you can reap the benefits of their nutritional content while enjoying their sweetness.

Sugar Substitutes

Sugar substitutes, or non-nutritive sweeteners (NNS), are commonly used to add a sweet taste to food or drinks with few to no calories. NNS can be categorized into two groups—artificial and natural. Artificial sweeteners and their brand names include aspartame (Equal), saccharin (Sweet'N Low), and sucralose (Splenda), and as their name implies, these sweeteners are artificially made through chemical processes. Natural NNS and their brand names include stevia leaf extract (Stevia in the Raw) and monk fruit extract (e.g., Splenda Monk Fruit). However, these natural sweeteners are often combined with chemical sweeteners, particularly erythritol.

Smart use of NNS can help reduce your intake of added sugar, contributing to a healthy body weight, which, in turn, may reduce the risk of chronic diseases like diabetes. Overall, the consensus seems to be that occasionally enjoying these sweeteners is perfectly okay. We tested a few of our recipes with monk fruit sweetener (which is often mixed with the NNS erythritol) and found that it tastes delicious and doesn't leave you with an unpleasant aftertaste, as stevia sometimes does. Check out the Appendix (page 249) to see our favorite monk fruit brands. If you prefer to avoid NNS, feel free to use your sweetener of choice. See the chart below for how to convert monk fruit to other sweeteners.

1 tablespoon Splenda Monk Fruit = 1 tablespoon honey, agave nectar, or maple syrup

1 tablespoon Splenda Monk Fruit = ½ teaspoon Truvia

1 tablespoon Splenda Monk Fruit = 1/16 teaspoon pure Stevia

Will All These Carbs Spike My Blood Sugar?

You may be hesitant to introduce high-carb meals into your diet, and we completely understand why. Maybe a banana sends your blood sugar soaring, or oatmeal causes an immediate spike in your glucose. Although a plant-based diet has the potential to reverse insulin resistance, the sudden re-introduction of carbohydrates into your diet may cause unwanted blood sugar spikes. But rest assured, we created these meal plans with this in mind. We carefully balanced the carb-to-fiber ratio in every recipe.

Plus, once you have committed to a more nutrient-dense, whole-food, plant-based eating pattern, you should be able to worry less about temporary rises in your blood sugar levels after meals. Over time—sometimes in a matter of days—the spikes will lessen as you regain insulin sensitivity. A clear sign that you are reversing insulin resistance and on your way to placing diabetes into remission is when your tolerance to carbohydrates improves, and you start seeing normal rises in your blood sugar after meals again.

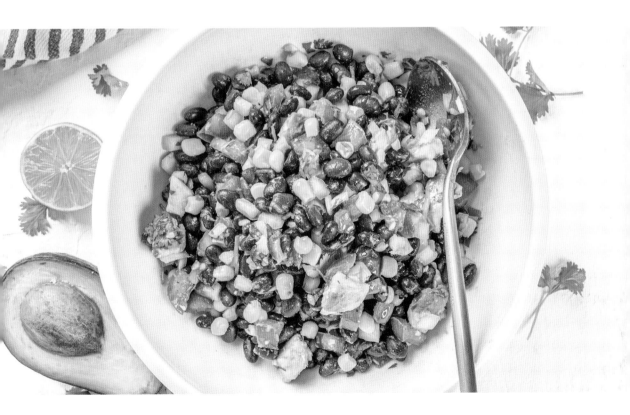

How Can I Reduce My Post-Meal Blood Sugar Levels?

If you currently experience elevated blood sugar levels after meals, or if you notice spikes after consuming some of the recipes in the meal plans, here are two tips that may help.

Include Unlimited Amounts of
Non-Starchy Vegetables with Meals

Vegetables, particularly non-starchy ones, are a great way to add bulk to your meals without causing a huge spike in blood glucose. These veggies have fewer carbohydrates than starchy vegetables but are still packed with vitamins, minerals, and fiber. Because they are nutrient-dense, meaning they are low in calories and high in nutrients, you can load up your plate with them. The more, the better! Refer back to Chapter 3 (page 39) for a list of common non-starchy veggies.

Aim for a 10- to 20-Minute Walk after Meals

Our muscles use glucose for energy, so if you experience a blood sugar spike after a meal, one of the best ways to bring it down is by activating your muscles. After a meal, glucose enters the bloodstream, causing blood sugar to rise. But when you exercise or move your muscles soon after eating, that glucose is absorbed by muscle tissue and eliminated from the bloodstream. Incorporating any sort of movement for at least 15 to 20 minutes after a meal works—walk, dance, bike ride, clean up your house, vacuum, walk up and down the stairs, or anything else to get your muscles moving. The longer you move, the greater effect it will have on your blood sugar. Moving after meals can also aid in digestion and improve your overall insulin sensitivity.

Is Soy Safe to Eat?

Absolutely! Unfortunately, soy receives a lot of bad press thanks to the media and their click-bait headlines and sensational reporting. Soy developed a bad reputation because it contains a compound called phytoestrogen. Because phytoestrogen has a similar structure to estrogen, people assume it exerts similar effects as estrogen (high levels of estrogen can disrupt reproductive processes). However, extensive research has shown that phytoestrogen does not act the same way as estrogen. In fact, soy has been associated with a decreased risk of prostate, GI, and breast cancer (among other types). The consumption of soy is also associated with a decreased risk of type 2 diabetes, and can help prevent osteoporosis, or the weakening of bones. Lastly, replacing animal proteins with soy can help to improve your cholesterol and body weight.

We encourage you to incorporate soy into your diet, as it's an excellent replacement for meat and provides an abundance of health benefits. Soy is found in tofu, edamame, soy milk, tempeh, soy sauce, and miso. If you've tried tofu before and are not a fan, we encourage you to give it another try—see page 48 for tips on using tofu in our recipes.

What if Beans Give me Gas?

Beans are a fantastic source of fiber to keep your gut microbiome happy and blood sugar in check. Some of the molecules in beans (like raffinose and oligosacchardies) pass through to our large intestine undigested. They serve as an excellent source of food for our good gut bacteria, and as the bacteria break it down through a process known as fermentation, gas is released.

The good news is that regularly eating beans increases your bodies' tolerance to them and reduces intestinal gas. So eat them regularly! In the meantime, here are five things you can do to avoid getting gassy with beans:

1) Go slow. Add beans slowly into your diet, starting with just a few table-spoons and build your way up.

2) If you are using dry beans, soak and rinse them well.

3) Cook beans until they are very soft.

4) Eat slowly and chew well with every bite.

5) If you are still experiencing gas, try taking a prebiotic supplement or digestive enzymes like Beano until your body becomes more tolerant.

Do I Need to Be Concerned with Salt/Sodium?

Sodium (the main ingredient in table salt) is an essential mineral we must obtain from our diets. But on average Americans tend to consume much more sodium than our bodies require, which can lead to high blood pressure, or hypertension, a major risk factor for heart disease and stroke.

We often associate sodium with only salt, but it's added to many foods you may not be aware of. Here are the top ten sources of sodium in the diet:

- Breads and rolls
- Pizza
- Sandwiches
- Cold cuts and cured meats (i.e., deli meats)
- Soups
- Burritos and tacos
- Savory snacks like chips, popcorn, and crackers
- Chicken (uncooked chicken is often injected with sodium as part of the poultry "plumping process")
- Cheese
- Eggs

The American Heart Association recommends keeping your sodium intake to between 1,500 and 2,300 milligrams per day, which is particularly important for people with diabetes because they already face a high risk of developing heart disease.

A whole-food, plant-based diet contains far less sodium than what the average American consumes. You'll notice we include salt in our recipes for flavor. If you're worried about your sodium intake, you can simply reduce the amount of salt used in the recipe, or skip the salt altogether and use other spices and herbs for flavor. (Check out our favorite salt alternatives in the Appendix, page 249.)

How Does Oil Factor Into These Recipes?

Most oils, with the exception of coconut and palm oil, contain healthy fats (unsaturated fat), which are excellent for heart health and insulin sensitivity. However, oils of any kind are high in calories since they are a concentrated fat from whole foods (avocado oil comes from avocados, olive oil comes from olives, etc.).

Let's compare the nutritional value of an oil versus its whole food source. While ½ cup of olives contains 86 calories, 8 grams of fat, 2 grams of fiber, and 1 gram of protein, ½ cup of olive oil contains almost 1,000 calories, over 100 grams of fat, and 0 grams of protein and fiber.

As you can see, ½ cup of olive oil contains significantly higher levels of fat and calories than ½ cup of olives.

Olive Oil vs. Olives

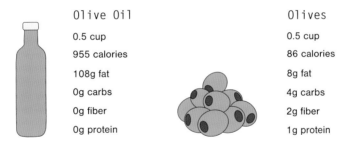

Olive Oil	Olives
0.5 cup	0.5 cup
955 calories	86 calories
108g fat	8g fat
0g carbs	4g carbs
0g fiber	2g fiber
0g protein	1g protein

To maximize the nutrient density of our meals, our recipes contain little to no oil and instead use whole-food sources of fat whenever possible. If you would like to use oil for sautéing or roasting, we recommend using olive oil cooking spray as this will help control the calories. But don't be fooled by the "zero calories" listed on cooking sprays. How might this be possible? The Food and Drug Administration allows food companies to claim zero calories if a serving contains less than five calories. Most cooking sprays have two calories per serving, and a serving size is a one-quarter-second spray. An average spray, though, is around four seconds, or 16 servings, resulting in 32 calories.

Here are some simple ways to reduce your oil intake during meal preparation:

- For sautéing: Use olive oil cooking spray, use a nonstick pan, or use water or vegetable stock, adding in a few tablespoons at a time and continuing to toss the food to prevent burning.

- For baking: Use mashed bananas, unsweetened applesauce, or a flax egg to replace the oil. These options will also add more nutrients and fiber to your baked goods.

- For roasting and steaming: Use olive oil cooking spray, or skip the oil altogether and stick with herbs and spices for flavor. Silicone baking mats are great for roasting, as they remove the need for oil and allow for an easy cleanup.

- For sauces: Puree beans with vegetables and add water or almond milk to liquefy them.

- For dressings: Blend whole nuts and seeds in a food processor for a creamy and nutrient-dense dressing.

How Will the Meal Plan Affect My Budget?

A common misconception about plant-based diets is that they are expensive, but this could not be further from the truth. Compared to the typical diet in the United States, a plant-based diet can reduce your food costs by over 30%. Unfortunately, healthier, minimally processed packaged foods (like whole-grain bread, cereals, crackers, etc.) are typically more expensive than their more processed counterparts, but this is more than balanced out by the savings you'll see from not purchasing animal-based products. While the individual food products listed in the Appendix may be pricier, your overall food costs will be lower with this dietary pattern.

What If I Have Food Allergies, I'm Gluten-Free, or I Have a Busy Schedule?

With every recipe, you'll find a variety of helpful tips. We always provide gluten-free options and ingredient-swap suggestions for the top allergens in the United States (which include tree nuts, peanuts, wheat, and soy). We also know that most people lead busy lives and can't always dedicate a lot of time to cooking, so with certain recipes, you'll see tips on saving time in the kitchen. (And of course, meal prepping on the weekend can help you save time as well.) You can also read the headnotes of each recipe to learn why we picked certain ingredients and how they can improve your blood sugar.

Do I Need to Follow the Meal Plan without Exception?

Not at all! Always start by making changes that you feel comfortable with. Making a diet change, no matter what it is, doesn't have to be a complete overhaul. Even if you don't follow the plan to the letter, you'll still gain tremendous health benefits by incorporating more plant-based meals into your diet.

If you want to start slow, try Meatless Mondays, which offers a manageable way to add more plant-based meals to your diet. Eliminating animal products one day a week makes the transition more doable. If a whole day is too overwhelming, start with one or two meals a day and work your way up from there. Continue adding meatless meals and days to further the transition to a more plant-based diet.

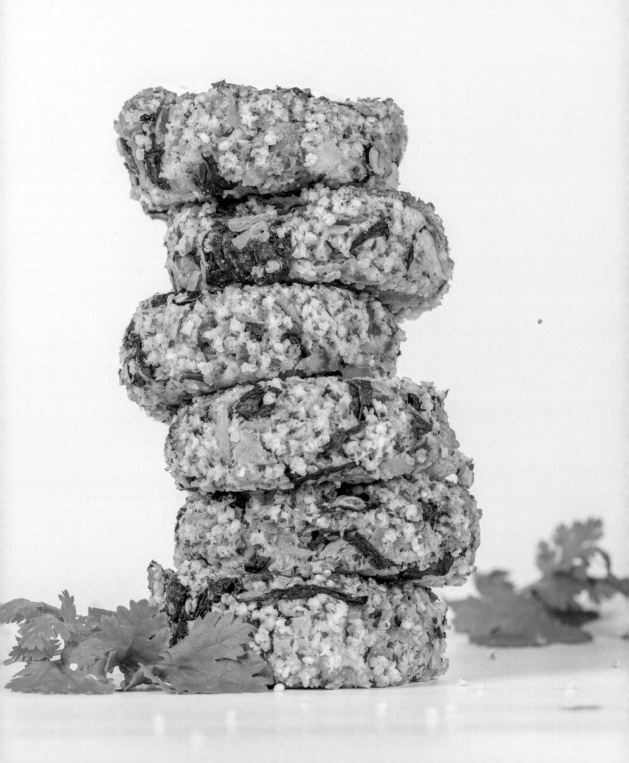

CHAPTER 5

The Meal Plan

Welcome to the meal plan! Our meal plans were designed for one person in mind, so if you are following them for yourself, follow the recipes as written (unless stated otherwise). For example, One-Pan Chickpeas with Rainbow Veggies serves 2 people but by making the entire recipe, it will serve as your lunch the next day. The White Bean and Lemon Kale Soup serves 6 people but by making the full recipe, you'll be able to freeze the leftovers and use it during another week (saving you time in the kitchen). For some meals, we've stated to cook "½ batch" (aka ½ the recipe), so that you don't end up with too many leftovers. If you plan to feed more than one, you can easily increase the quantities of the recipes but you will also have to increase the quantities on the grocery list.

Don't be surprised that there is plenty of cooking involved, but we've set up the meal plans and meal prep sections to minimize your time spent in the kitchen. For example, the extra servings you cook at dinner will serve as lunch the next day. Remember, though, you'll need plenty of food storage containers and Ziploc or reusable bags to store your food.

If you're new to cooking, don't feel intimidated. These recipes are easy to follow, and as you become more familiar with chopping and other meal prep activities, the time you spend in the kitchen will decrease. Plus, Week 1 shopping list is long because it includes staple items that are used throughout the four-week program; you may already have many of these (spices, nut butters, etc.) on hand.

The meal plans only include breakfast, lunch, and dinner, so incorporate snacks and desserts as you see fit. Not everyone enjoys snacks, and not everyone prefers dessert at night. We've left it for you to decide if and when. If you eat breakfast early and feel hungry again mid-morning, then have a snack. If you prefer to have a snack or something sweet after dinner, that's fine too! We've made the meal plans flexible so that you can tailor them to your hunger level and schedule.

To minimize food waste, we offer ideas for using leftover ingredients for snacks, side dishes, and recipe add-ins as well. We also provide dessert options for you to choose from.

Our grocery lists and meal plans are set up so that you shop and meal prep over the weekend; however, feel free to meal prep any day that works for your schedule. Please note, the ingredients for each Sunday's dinner have been included in the list of ingredients for the following week, so when you grocery shop and meal prep over the weekend, you'll have fresh ingredients to use to make that Sunday's dinner.

Week 1

Welcome to week 1 of the meal plan! You're on the path to seeing improvements in your blood sugar while enjoying carbs. If you feel comfortable doing so, track your fasting blood sugar daily (or at least a few times a week) to measure your progress. Once you've gathered 20 to 30 data points, you can hopefully identify a pattern. A downward trend reflects your hard work coming to fruition.

This week will contain meals with a lower carb-to-fiber ratio to help minimize blood sugar spikes as you start this new dietary pattern. Remember, if you experience spikes after eating, the best way to bring them down is through 20 minutes of light exercise, such as a walk around the block, a bike ride, dancing, or tidying up around the house. The longer you move, the greater its effect on your blood sugar. For each recipe in the meal plan, follow the recipe in the cookbook as is, unless stated otherwise.

Grocery List

Fruit

- 12 ounces berries (1½ cups), plus more for snacks, if desired
- 4 pieces fruit of choice, plus more for snacks, if desired
- 1 medium avocado
- 2 apples
- 1 lime
- 1 lemon

Vegetables

- Baby spinach (4 cups), or dark leafy green of choice
- Broccoli (2 cups)
- 3 carrots
- 1 head cauliflower
- Celery
- 1 large carton cherry tomatoes (2 cups)
- 3 garlic bulbs
- 1 bunch green onions
- Kale (1 cup)
- Purple cabbage (1 cup)
- 1 head romaine lettuce leaves
- 2 red bell peppers
- 2 yellow bell peppers
- 2 plum tomatoes
- 1 red onion
- 2 yellow onions
- 2 zucchini (or 1 package of pre-made zoodles)

Whole Grains

- Corn tortillas (4 tortillas)
- Whole-grain bread
- Brown rice

Proteins

- 2 (14-ounce) packages tofu, extra firm
- 2 (15-ounce) cans chickpeas
- 1 (15-ounce) can white beans
- 1 (15-ounce) can pinto beans
- 1 (16-ounce) bag dry green or brown lentils
- 1 (16-ounce) bag dry red lentils
- Protein powder
- Hummus (if making home-made Oil-Free Hummus, find ingredients on page 226)

Boxed and Canned

- 1 (15-ounce) can light coconut milk
- 1 (6-ounce) can tomato paste
- 1 (32-ounce) carton vegetable stock

Nuts, Seeds, and Spices

- Nut or seed butter
- Walnuts
- Cashews
- Chia seeds
- Salt
- Black pepper
- Cayenne pepper
- Chili powder
- Cinnamon
- Cumin
- Curry powder
- Garam masala
- Garlic powder
- Onion powder
- Dried oregano
- Red pepper flakes

Condiments

- Balsamic vinegar
- Capers
- Less-sodium soy sauce, tamari, or coconut aminos
- Vegan mayonnaise
- Nutritional yeast
- Vanilla extract
- Monk fruit sweetener

Non-Dairy

- Non-dairy milk of choice, plain and unsweetened
- Non-dairy yogurt of choice, plain and unsweetened

Frozen

- Frozen peas

Meal Prep

- Prep and divide 3 batches of Creamy Chia Seed Puddings.
- Prep a batch of the Creamy Balsamic Vinaigrette.
  - *For Mix-and-Match Mason Jar Salad and One-Pan Chickpeas with Rainbow Veggies*
- Make 3–4 cups of cooked brown rice (cheaper option) OR buy a few bags of pre-cooked brown rice (quicker option).
  - *For Mix and Match Mason Jar Salad, Curried Lentils (if desired), and Sticky Veggie Fried Rice*
- Cut half of the cauliflower head into florets and process the other half into cauliflower rice.
  - *For Curried Lentils (florets) and Sticky Veggie Fried Rice (cauliflower rice)*
- Dice the carrots.
  - *For Lentil "No Meat" Sauce and Sticky Veggie Fried Rice*
- Dice the yellow onions.
  - *For various meals*
- Shred the cabbage.
  - *For Mix-and-Match Mason Jason Salad and Sticky Veggie Fried Rice*
- Cut the broccoli into florets (or buy pre-cut broccoli), slice a yellow bell pepper, and cube the red onion.
  - *For One-Pan Chickpeas with Rainbow Veggies*
- Spiralize the zucchini into noodles (or buy pre-made zoodles).
  - *For Lentil "No Meat" Sauce*
- Slice yellow and red bell peppers.
  - *For Pinto Bean Fajitas*

	Monday	Tuesday	Wednesday
Breakfast	Creamy Chia Seed Pudding (page 108)	Protein-Packed Avocado Toast (page 107)	Creamy Chia Seed Pudding
Lunch	Mix-and-Match Mason Jar Salad (page 70)	Curried Lentils with Kale and Cauliflower + ½ cup brown rice, if desired	Sticky Veggie Fried R
Dinner	½ batch Curried Lentils with Kale and Cauliflower (page 158) + ½ cup brown rice, if desired	Sticky Veggie Fried Rice (page 161)	One-Pan Chickpea with Rainbow Veggies (page 168) + 1 batch of Cream Balsamic Vinaigrett

Thursday	Friday	Saturday	Sunday
Protein-Packed Avocado Toast	Creamy Chia Seed Pudding	Tofu Veggie Scramble (page 114) + 1 serving of fruit + 1–2 slices whole-grain bread	Tofu Veggie Scramble + 1 serving of fruit + 1–2 slices whole-grain bread
e-Pan Chickpeas with Rainbow Veggies	Lentil "No Meat" Sauce + Zucchini Noodles	Chickpea Toona Lettuce Wraps (page 139)	Chickpea Toona Lettuce Wraps
ntil "No Meat" Sauce + Zucchini Noodles (page 220)	Pinto Bean Fajitas (page 172)	Pinto Bean Fajitas	

Mix-and-Match Mason Jar Salad

Use leftover ingredients from meal prep to create Monday's lunch:

- Brown rice (~½ cup)

- Leftover white beans and pinto beans (~¾-1 cup)

- Leftover veggies like the cherry tomatoes, broccoli, cabbage, kale/spinach, and avocado

- Use Creamy Balsamic Vinaigrette (page 224) for dressing

Snacks

- Use extra celery for dipping in peanut butter.

- Use leftover broccoli, bell peppers, and celery for dipping in hummus.

- Combine extra fruit and ¼ cup of nuts.

- Combine leftover yogurt with fruit, nut butter, and 1/2 scoop protein powder, if desired.

Use Up Leftovers

- Top extra vegetables with Creamy Balsamic Vinaigrette to create side salads for your dishes.

- Use romaine lettuce, avocado, tomatoes, and shredded cabbage for taco toppings. Use romaine leaves as additional "tortillas."

- Use kale, spinach, and romaine to add extra greens to any meals.

- Freeze leftover spinach, kale, onions, bell peppers, and broccoli and use them in smoothies, soups, or stir-fries.

- Use leftover coconut milk in coffee or tea.

- Add lime and lemon slices to your water.

Desserts, if desired (not included in grocery list)

- Chocolate Chia Pudding (page 208)
- Grilled Peaches with Cinnamon (page 213)
- Chocolate-Covered Strawberries (page 217)

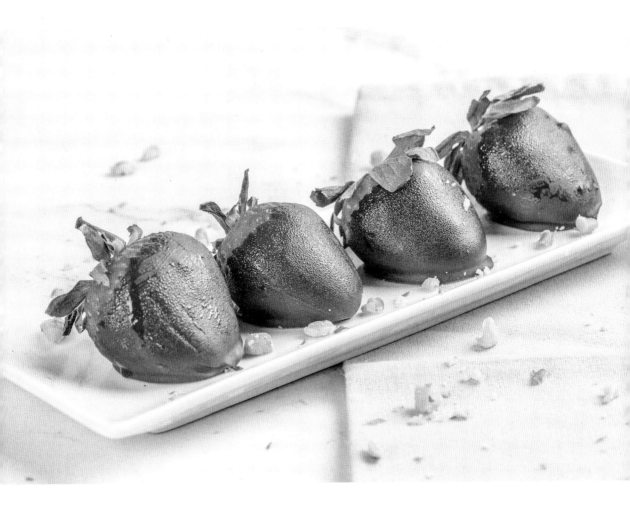

Week 2

Welcome to week 2 of the meal plan. We hope you enjoyed week 1 and didn't find it too overwhelming. Meal prepping and cooking become easier each week. Some people may already notice a decline in their blood sugar by this point. If you haven't yet, or have seen higher than your baseline readings, these are all normal responses. Remember, you're actively working on reversing the root cause—insulin resistance—and for some people, it takes longer than others. Some people may even see an initial increase before it starts to come down, but don't get discouraged. The best way to succeed is to stay committed and motivated.

For this week's meal prep, pull out your high-speed blender or food processor, because you'll be prepping many dressings and sauces! The good news is that it's quick and easy to do.

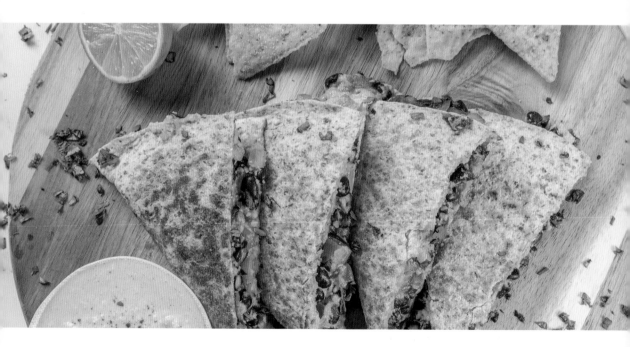

Grocery List

Fruit

- 3 avocados (two ripe, one green)
- 5 pieces fresh fruit of choice, plus more for snacks, if desired
- 1 lemon
- 1 lime

Vegetables

- 1–2 bags baby spinach (5½ cups)
- Basil (¼ cup)
- Broccoli (1 head)
- 2 carrots
- Celery
- Cilantro (⅓ cup)
- 3 garlic bulbs
- 1 thumb-size piece ginger
- Kale (4 cups)
- Mushrooms (1 cup)
- Parsley (2 cups)
- 3 red bell peppers
- 1 bag romaine lettuce (3 heads)
- 3 tomatoes
- 1 white onion
- 3 yellow onions

Whole Grains

- 1 (15-ounce) can corn (or 1 bag frozen corn)
- Whole-grain bread
- Whole-wheat tortillas
- Quinoa
- Steel-cut oats

Proteins

- 3 (15-ounce) cans white beans, any kind
- 3 (15-ounce) cans chickpeas
- 2 (15-ounce) cans black beans
- 1 (8-ounce) package tempeh
- 1 (14-ounce) package tofu, extra firm

Canned and Boxed

- 2 (32-ounce) cartons vegetable stock

Nuts, Seeds, and Spices

- Ground flaxseed
- Brazil nuts (or almonds)
- Cashews
- Tahini

- Paprika
- Ground turmeric
- Dried dill
- Dried parsley

Condiments

- Apple cider vinegar
- Dijon mustard

Frozen

- 1 bag frozen blueberries (2 cups)

Non-dairy

- 2 cartons non-dairy milk of choice, plain and unsweetened

Leftovers You May Already Have on Hand

- Brown lentils
- Capers
- Chia seeds
- Less-sodium soy sauce, tamari, or coconut aminos

- Nutritional yeast
- Vanilla extract
- Monk fruit sweetener
- Protein powder

Meal Prep

- Cook White Bean and Lemon Kale Soup; divide and freeze leftovers.

- Prep Blueberry Steel-Cut Oats and Eggless "Egg" Cups.

- Make Cashew Nacho "Cheese" Sauce, Tahini Caesar Dressing, and Green Goddess Drizzle.

- Make Nutty "Cheese" Topper and 2 batches of Crispy Chickpeas (any style)
  - *For Chickpea "Caesar" Salad and for snacking (2nd batch of crispy chickpeas)*

- Dice onions
  - *Multiple meals*

- Chop broccoli into florets (or buy pre-cut broccoli).
  - *For Teriyaki Tempeh and Broccoli*

- Dice 1 red bell pepper
  - *For Eggless "Egg" Cups and Black Bean Quesadillas*

- Chop romaine (leave some leaves whole for Black Bean and Corn Salad)
  - *For Chickpea "Caesar" Salad*

	Sunday	Monday	Tuesday	Wednesday
Breakfast		Meal Prep Blueberry Steel-Cut Oats (page 110)	3 Eggless "Egg" Cups (page 119) + 1 serving of fruit + 1–2 slices whole-grain bread	Meal Prep Blueber Steel-Cut Oats
Lunch		White Bean and Lemon Kale Soup + 1–2 slices whole-grain bread	Stuffed Peppers with Lentils	Chickpea "Caesa Salad Wrap (serve in a whole-whea tortilla)
Dinner	White Bean and Lemon Kale Soup (page 137) + 1-2 slices whole-grain bread	½ batch Stuffed Peppers with Lentils (page 176)	½ batch Chickpea "Caesar" Salad Wrap (page 153; served in a whole-wheat tortilla)	½ batch Black Be and Corn Salad (page 153; page 1 served in lettuc wraps with Gree Goddess Drizzle

Thursday	Friday	Saturday	Sunday
Eggless "Egg" Cups 1 serving of fruit + 2 slices whole-grain bread	Meal Prep Blueberry Steel-Cut Oats	3 Eggless "Egg" Cups + 1 serving of fruit + 1–2 slices whole-grain bread	Meal Prep Blueberry Steel- Cut Oats
ack Bean and Corn ad (served in lettuce wraps with Green Goddess Drizzle)	Teriyaki Tempeh and Broccoli Stir-Fry	Creamy Chickpea Avocado Sandwich (page 142) + 1 piece of fruit	Creamy Chickpea Avocado Sandwich + 1 piece of fruit
Teriyaki Tempeh nd Broccoli Stir-Fry (page 178)	Black Bean Quesadillas with Cashew Nacho "Cheese" Sauce (page 184)	Black Bean Quesadillas with Cashew Nacho "Cheese" Sauce	

Snacks

- The second batch of Crispy Chickpeas will serve as a snack for the week.

- Use extra celery for dipping in peanut butter.

- Use unused broccoli, bell peppers, and celery for dipping in leftover dressings or sauces.

- Combine extra fruit with ¼ cup of nuts.

- Use leftover avocado to make Avocado and Tomato Toast (page 192).

- Throw leftover beans together with tomato, onion, and cilantro and top it with any dressing or sauce to make a bean salad.

Use Up Leftovers

- Divide and freeze leftover White Bean and Lemon Kale Soup (this will be used again for week 4).

- Use kale, spinach, and romaine to add extra greens to any meals.

- Freeze leftover spinach, kale, onions, bell peppers, broccoli, and ginger and use them for smoothies, soups, or stir-fries.

- Add ginger, lemon, and lime slices to your water.

Desserts, if desired (not included in grocery list)

- Epic Rainbow Fruit Salad (page 211)

- Fudgy Brownies (page 214)

- Chocolate-Covered Snicker Dates (page 206)

Week 3

Congratulations, you're halfway through the meal plan! Meal prep for this week's meal plan is only a few steps and should be completed relatively quickly. We hope you're starting to see improvements in your fasting blood sugar. Many people also report seeing a change in weight at this mark as well. However, don't get discouraged if you're not seeing any improvements yet; this is also normal. Keep up the great work, and the results will come.

Grocery List

Fruit

- 3 ripe bananas
- 1 carton blueberries (½ cup)
- 1 lime
- 1 lemon
- Fruit of choice for snacks, if desired

Vegetables

- Baby spinach (4 cups)
- Basil (2 cups)
- Broccoli (½ cup)
- 1 carrot
- Cherry tomatoes (2½ cups)
- 1 cucumber
- 1 large eggplant
- 3 garlic bulbs
- 1 pumpkin (or three 15-ounce cans pumpkin puree)
- 1 head purple cabbage (½ cups shredded)
- 1 red bell pepper
- 1 sprig rosemary
- 1 plum tomato
- 2 yellow onions
- 1 red onion

Whole Grains

- Whole-grain bread
- Whole-grain cereal
- Whole-wheat pita
- Brown rice noodles
- 1 (16-ounce) box whole-wheat penne
- Rolled oats

Proteins

- 1 (15-ounce) can black beans
- 2 (15-ounce) cans chickpeas
- 2 (15-ounce) cans white beans
- 2 (14-ounce) packages tofu, extra firm
- 1 (16-ounce) box bean pasta

Canned and Boxed

- 1 (32-ounce) carton vegetable stock
- 1 (15-ounce) can of tomato sauce
- 1 (15-ounce) can light coconut milk

Nuts, Seeds, and Spices

- Pine nuts
- Peanuts

Condiments

- 1 (24-ounce) jar pasta sauce (if making home made Fresh Basil Pasta Sauce, find ingredients on page 224)
- Sriracha
- Baking powder
- Rice vinegar

Frozen

- 1 bag blueberries (2 cups)
- 1 bag edamame (1 to 2 cups)

Non-dairy

- Non-dairy milk of choice, plain and unsweetened
- Non-dairy yogurt, plain and unsweetened

Leftovers You May Already Have on Hand

- Chia seeds
- Corn tortillas
- Balsamic vinegar
- Less-sodium soy sauce, tamari, or coconut aminos
- Tahini
- Nut or seed butter
- Protein powder
- Nutritional yeast
- Vanilla extract

Meal Prep

- Make the Roasted Pumpkin and White Bean Soup; divide into containers and freeze leftovers.

- Make a batch of Blueberry Breakfast Muffins.

- Make a batch of the Herbed "Ricotta" Filling.

- Make a batch of Basil Spinach Pesto.

- On Wednesday morning, move frozen leftover White Bean and Lemon Kale Soup into the fridge.

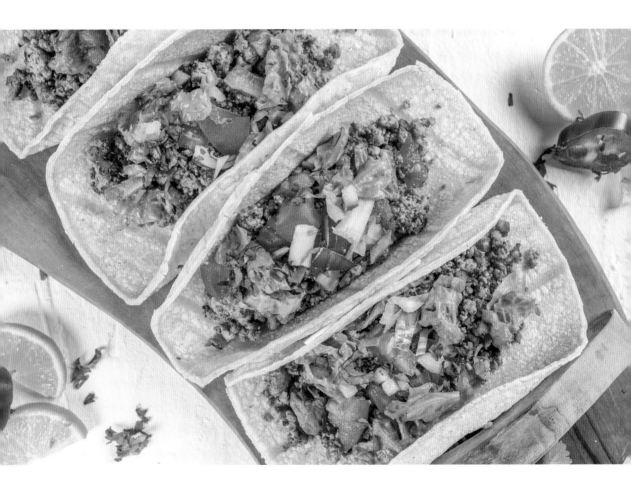

	Sunday	Monday	Tuesday	Wednesday
Breakfast		2 Blueberry Breakfast Muffins (page 126) + 1 tablespoon nut butter	Berry Vanilla Yogurt Parfait (page 115)	2 Blueberry Breakfast Muffins + 1 tablespoon nut butter
Lunch		Roasted Pumpkin and White Bean Soup + 1-2 slices whole-grain bread	Penne Pesto with Spinach and Cherry Tomatoes	Tofu Crumble Taco
Dinner	Roasted Pumpkin and White Bean Soup (page 131) + 1-2 slices whole-grain bread	½ batch Penne Pesto with Spinach and Cherry Tomatoes (page 166)	Tofu Crumble Tacos (page 165)	White Bean and Lemon Kale Soup 1-2 slices of whole grain bread

Thursday	Friday	Saturday	Sunday
Berry Vanilla Yogurt Parfait	2 Blueberry Breakfast Muffins + 1 tablespoon nut butter	"Ricotta" Toast with Cherry Tomatoes (page 122)	2 Blueberry Breakfast Muffins + 1 tablespoon nut butter
hite Bean and Lemon ale Soup + 1–2 slices f whole-grain bread	Eggplant "Ricotta" Roll-Ups + ½ cup bean pasta, if desired	Chopped Salad Pita Pockets (page 141)	Chopped Salad Pita Pockets
Eggplant "Ricotta" Roll-Ups (page 175) th ½ cup bean pasta, if desired	½ batch Veggie Pad Thai Noodles (page 183)	Veggie Pad Thai Noodles	

Snacks

- Use leftover bell peppers, broccoli, and any other veggies for dipping in unused hummus.

- Combine extra blueberries with ¼ cup nuts.

- Spread extra pesto on whole-wheat toast or crackers.

- Combine leftover yogurt with fruit, nut butter, and ½ scoop protein powder.

- Combine unused beans, cabbage, and onions with any leftover dressing or sauce to enjoy as a bean salad.

- Make the Garlic Spiced Edamame (page 188) using leftover edamame.

Use Up Leftovers

- Use leftover tomato and shredded cabbage as taco toppings.

- Add unused greens to any meals.

- Freeze leftover spinach, onions, bell peppers, and broccoli and use in soups or stir-fries.

- Add extra lemon and lime slices to water.

Desserts, if desired (not included in grocery list)

- Slow Cooker Cinnamon Applesauce (page 212)

- No-Sugar-Added Ice Cream (page 202)

Week 4

Congratulations on reaching the last week of the meal plan. You're almost there! If you've made it this far, you're well on your way to a life free of diabetes. Hopefully, you have a good grasp on how to eat more plant-based foods and can continue this way of eating beyond the four weeks. If you notice your fasting blood sugar values in the low 100s mg/dL (5.6 mmol/L) for two straight weeks, you should consult your physician about lowering your medications. As a reminder, progress is rarely linear so don't let minor setbacks discourage you from your goals. Consistency is key!

Grocery List

Fruit

- 1 avocado
- 3 ripe bananas
- 1 carton blueberries (1½ cups)
- 2 pieces fruit of choice, plus more for snacks, if desired
- 1 lemon
- 1 lime

Vegetables

- Arugula (2 cups)
- Broccoli (½ cup)
- 1 carrot
- 1 small bunch of cilantro
- 2 garlic bulbs
- 1 bunch green onions
- 1 jalapeño pepper
- Mushrooms (1½ cups)
- 1 small bunch of parsley
- 2 red bell peppers
- 1 yellow bell pepper
- 1 red onion
- 3 sweet potatoes
- 2 yellow onions
- 2 zucchini

Whole Grains

- Whole-wheat bread crumbs
- Farro
- Millet
- Quinoa
- 1 (15-ounce) can corn (or 1 bag frozen corn)
- Whole-grain bread

Proteins

- 4 (15-ounce) cans black beans
- 2 (15-ounce) cans chickpeas
- 1 (15-ounce) can pinto beans
- 1 (14-ounce) package tofu, extra firm
- Bean pasta

Canned and Boxed

- 1 (32-ounce) carton vegetable stock
- 2 (15-ounce) cans diced tomatoes
- 1 (24-ounce) jar pasta sauce
- Cornstarch

Nuts, Seeds, and Spices

- Old Bay seasoning

Frozen

- Frozen strawberries (4 cups)

Non-dairy

- Non-dairy milk of choice, plain and unsweetened

Leftovers You May Already Have on Hand

- Rolled oats (3 cups)
- Vanilla extract
- Monk fruit sweetener
- Baking powder
- Cashews
- Chia seeds
- Ground flax seed
- Walnuts
- Corn tortillas
- Frozen cauliflower rice (1 cup)
- Nut butter
- Tomato paste
- Apple cider vinegar
- Balsamic vinegar
- Vegan mayonnaise
- Nutritional yeast
- Protein powder

Meal Prep

- Cook the Hearty 3-Bean Chili; divide into containers and freeze leftovers.

- Make 3 batches of the PB&J Overnight Oats.

- Make a batch of the No-Sugar-Added Berry Chia Jam.

- Make a batch of the Creamy Balsamic Vinaigrette.

- Peel and freeze 2 of the bananas.

  - *For Smoothies*

- Chop the sweet potatoes and cook the millet.

  - *For Roasted Sweet Potato Salad with Arugula and Millet and Sweet Potato Black Bean Quinoa Bake*

- Slice the red onions and chop the broccoli into florets.

  - *For Pasta Primavera*

- Make the Mushroom Black Bean Burger patties and freeze them.

- On Tuesday morning, move the leftover frozen Roasted Pumpkin and White Bean Soup into the fridge.

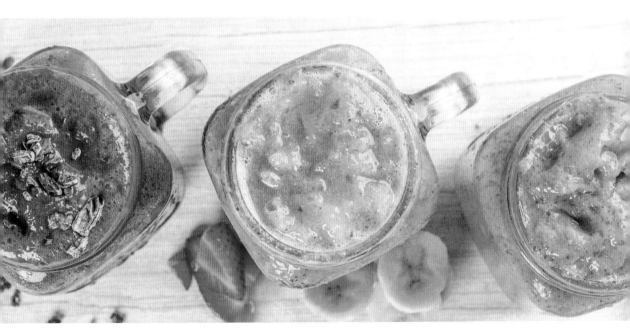

	Sunday	Monday	Tuesday	Wednesday
Breakfast		PB&J Overnight Oats (page 125)	Strawberry Banana Smoothie (page 116) + 1 scoop protein powder	PB&J Overnight O
Lunch		Hearty 3-Bean Chili	Roasted Sweet Potato Salad with Arugula and Millet	Roasted Pumpki and White Bean So + 1-2 slices of who grain bread
Dinner	Hearty 3-Bean Chili (page 134)	½ batch Roasted Sweet Potato Salad with Arugula and Millet (page 145)	Roasted Pumpkin and White Bean Soup (page 131) + 1-2 slices of whole-grain bread	Sweet Potato Blac Bean Quinoa Bak (page 159)

Thursday	Friday	Saturday	Sunday
Strawberry Banana Smoothie + 1 scoop protein powder	PB&J Overnight Oats	Protein Banana Pancakes (page 121) + 1 batch of No-Sugar-Added Berry Jam	Protein Banana Pancakes
Sweet Potato Black Bean Quinoa Bake	Breaded Tofu "Fish" Fingers	½ batch Black Bean Farro Salad (page 150)	Black Bean Farro Salad
Breaded Tofu "Fish" Fingers (page 173)	½ batch Pasta Primavera (page 182)	Pasta Primavera	Mushroom Black Bean Burgers (page 162)

Snacks

- Use leftover broccoli, bell peppers, and carrots for dipping in extra Creamy Balsamic Vinaigrette.

- Combine extra fruit with ¼ cup nuts.

- Use leftover avocado to make Avocado and Tomato Toast (page 192)

- Combine unused beans, cilantro, bell peppers, and onions with leftover dressing or sauce to enjoy as a bean salad.

Use Up Leftovers

- Use arugula and avocado for taco toppings.

- Use extra greens for any meals, especially lunches.

- Use extra veggies to make side salads.

- Freeze leftover onions, bell peppers, and broccoli and use them in smoothies, soups, or stir-fries.

- Add lemon and lime slices to your water.

Desserts, if desired (not included in grocery list)

- Fruity Sorbet (page 205)

- Chocolate Date Balls (page 203)

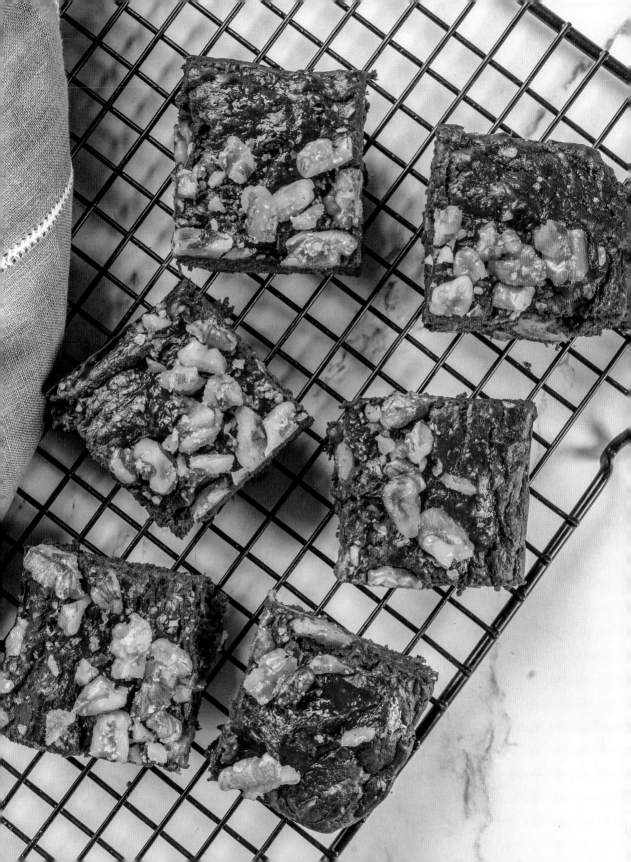

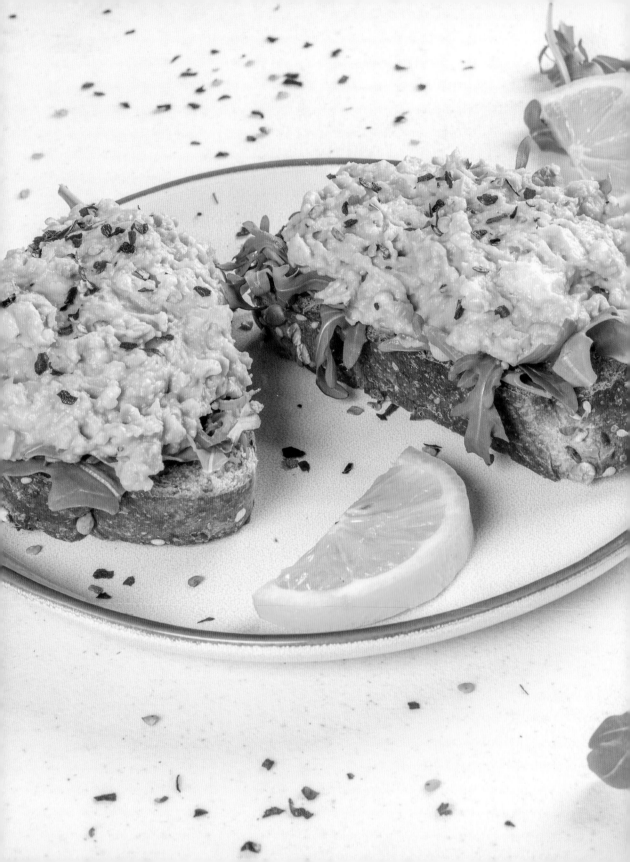

CHAPTER 6

Beyond the Four Weeks

Type 2 Diabetes Remission: A Possibility Within Your Reach

If you've been following our meal plans and staying active over the past four weeks, you're likely seeing a downward trend in your blood sugar. Trends are more reliable indicators of progress than individual blood sugar readings. For this reason, we recommend checking your fasting blood glucose levels daily (or at least a few times a week) and keeping a detailed log of those values. Once you've gathered 20 to 30 data points, you can hopefully identify a pattern. A downward trend reflects your hard work coming to fruition. Keep up the great work!

Remember that four weeks is a relatively short time to see significant results. We suggest giving yourself ten to sixteen weeks of consistent effort with our approach. Anecdotal data from our coaching program suggests that members see satisfactory results and eliminate (or reduce) medications after three to six months. We recommend informing your physician before starting any lifestyle change, especially when taking prescription medications, so they can guide you through the de-prescription process.

Putting type 2 diabetes into remission takes time and consistency. But the relief you'll feel knowing that your health is no longer declining is indescribable; just read about our member Meghan's incredible experience:

> *"When I began this program, I was diagnosed with type 2 diabetes and my A1c was 10.7%. Today, I went to my endocrinologist and found out that my A1c is now 5.7%. YES, this program has changed my life forever! I was hoping to hear that my A1c held steady at 6.2% from my last appointment three months ago, but this was the most elating news I could have ever dreamed of. I'm no longer diabetic in any way, shape, or form. . . all my fears of the many complications that come with type 2 diabetes are now gone. I've been floating on air all day. As my doctor said, 'You've given yourself the gift of health and all of the potential complications you will now not have to deal with.' I'm so incredibly grateful to have found Diana and Jose because they saved my life."*

As evidenced by the testimonial above, it took Meghan a few months to drop her A1c from 10.7% to 5.7%, but with perseverance and consistency, she did it! Other members join our program hoping to reduce or eliminate their need for medications—a common outcome. Read what our member Hugo shared in our program's community forum:

> *"Good morning, everyone! I wanted to share this post with all of you in the hopes that it might encourage some of you on this type 2 diabetes journey. I was diagnosed with T2D at the end of February with an A1c of 12% and started the program on March 2. I was on two diabetes meds, two cholesterol meds, and one for high blood pressure. Within five to six weeks, I had gradually stopped all medications and have been off medications ever since. I redid my blood work this week, and my A1c has dropped within normal to 5.6%!!! I am so very grateful to have found this program, and for all the help and guidance I received from Jose and Diana. They've made a plant-based eater out of me!!!"*

Living without medications is achievable with our approach. Again, we can't stress the importance enough of going through a de-prescription process with the help of your physician, who will provide guidance and close monitoring. If you notice your fasting blood sugar values in the low 100s mg/dL (5.6 mmol/L) for two straight weeks, you should consult with your physician about lowering your medications.

Reincorporating Animal-Based Foods into Your Diet

The Adventist Health Study 2 examined the prevalence of type 2 diabetes among nearly 61,000 people. The researchers found that the higher the consumption of animal-based foods, the higher the risk of diabetes. Vegans (100% plant-based eaters) experienced the lowest prevalence of diabetes (2.9%), with the percentage consistently rising with every dietary pattern that included more animal foods—lacto-ovo (3.2%), pescatarian (4.8%), semi-vegetarian (6.1%), and nonvegetarian (7.6%). This study suggests that the more closely we can follow a plant-based diet, the less likely we may be to suffer from type 2 diabetes. However, this doesn't mean that animal-based foods must be completely off-limits.

Hugo, from the testimonial on the previous page, wanted to reintroduce animal-based foods into his diet. After following a plant-based, whole-food diet for several months, achieving normal blood sugar, and eliminating all his medications, he felt ready. Keeping most of his diet composed of whole-food, plant-based meals, Hugo added fish a few times a week and red meat a few times a month. He continued to monitor his fasting blood sugar levels as he added these foods to find a healthy balance that worked for him. He has successfully kept his blood sugar within the normal range. Tolerance for saturated fat from animal products will differ, so as you reintroduce animal products into your diet, track your fasting blood sugar and weight to monitor your insulin resistance. If you notice an upward trend in your fasting blood sugar, consider cutting back on these foods.

Dealing with Social Situations

Social situations can be difficult to navigate when trying to stay healthy and manage diabetes. But remember, the foods you eat consistently and regularly will have the most significant impact on your health and diabetes management—this is why the 80/20 approach works so well. If 80% of your diet consists of plant-based, whole foods then the remaining 20% offers wiggle room for more processed foods and animal-based options.

It's easy to overindulge in social situations. To prevent overeating, pay attention to your fullness cues and try to stop eating when full. Avoid eating mindlessly due to boredom or distraction, and cease eating before abdominal discomfort sets in. Including high-fiber carbohydrates (whole grains), lean protein (preferably from plant-based sources like legumes), and vegetables and/or fruit with every meal and snack can also help ensure you eat satiating meals that will fill you up and keep you full. We hope the recipes in this book have given you ideas on combining these food groups to create filling and satisfying dishes. Enjoy yourself in social situations, but focus on portion control, choosing satiating meals, and stopping when you feel full. Lastly, sometimes we overdo it, and that's okay. If this does happen, don't hyper-focus on it or punish yourself—just move on!

Important Factors for Long-Term Success and How We Can Help

We have a mission of giving millions of people access to proper diabetes education and coaching. The current healthcare system doesn't have the capacity to deliver this. In traditional diabetes care, patients are given little education or coaching, even though evidence confirms that coaching significantly improves glycemic control and HbA1c in patients with type 2 diabetes. What's more, virtual coaching aids glycemic control, promotes behavioral change, and offers valuable psychosocial support, especially given its immediate, real-time availability.

We've built a platform that offers a variety of programs focused on core elements that improve diabetes outcomes. While nutrition is one of the most important factors for putting diabetes into remission, it's not the only one. Our programs examine in detail the nutrition topics covered in this book, provide many more customized recipes and meal plans, and explore other lifestyle factors of importance in overcoming diabetes. Read on to learn how and why these other lifestyle factors are equally important in your journey to overcome diabetes.

Find Your Community

Research shows that joining a group program facilitates behavior change and helps with accountability, especially in the long term. Group programs create a more supportive environment where members feel less alone, regardless of their challenges. Finding your community through a group program can lead to better diabetes outcomes compared to managing diabetes by yourself. Members of these programs experience significant decreases in HbA1c, improved diet, and better blood glucose regulation. The majority of our programs offer access to a tight-knit community where you'll find support, accountability, and encouragement from others embarking on a similar journey.

Get Support from a Multidisciplinary Healthcare Team

A multidisciplinary diabetes team includes a group of different healthcare providers working together to support the needs of a person with diabetes. The benefits of working with a multidisciplinary team include:[74]

- Access to experts in various areas of diabetes management
- Better glycemic control
- Increased patient follow-up
- Greater patient satisfaction
- Lower risk for diabetes complications
- Improved quality of life
- Reduced hospitalizations
- Decreased healthcare costs

We've built a multidisciplinary team of registered dietitians, certified diabetes care and education specialists, exercise physiologists, and endocrinologists to provide optimal care for our members. This multidisciplinary approach provides a unique edge. Our dietitians support you with advice on nutrition, diet, and other lifestyle factors such as sleep and stress. They keep you accountable for your goals and help you establish long-lasting habits. Our exercise physiologists create custom exercise routines for you, while our endocrinologists work with you to lower your prescription medications as your blood sugar improves.

Stay Physically Active

Physical activity can lead to better mood and sleep, reduced depression, higher bone density, weight loss, and improved quality of life. But above all, it plays a crucial role in diabetes management. Even just a 15-minute walk can have an impact on your blood sugar.

Muscle is the most abundant and metabolically active organ in our body—meaning it requires a lot of energy (glucose) during periods of both exercise and rest. Therefore, the more muscle you have, the more glucose your muscles will use for energy. Our liver and brain also use large amounts of glucose, but unlike our muscles, we can't directly manipulate these organs to use more energy. On the other hand, muscles can be encouraged to use more glucose through exercise. Regular physical activity lowers blood glucose levels, improves glycemic control, and increases insulin sensitivity. And the opposite is also true: low muscle strength and tone are both associated with a higher incidence of insulin resistance and type 2 diabetes.

Exercise is an essential component of our programs. Our more basic programs include exercise videos and routines designed to help you maximize glucose absorption. In our more customized programs, our exercise physiologists design specific routines that fit your needs, preferences, and abilities.

Reduce Stress and Establish Healthy Sleep Patterns

Stress and sleep also play an important role in blood glucose regulation. When chronically stressed, our bodies respond by secreting "fight or flight" hormones such as cortisol and adrenaline. These hormones stimulate the release of glucose from the liver, supplementing the amount already in the bloodstream. And to ensure that blood glucose levels remain elevated, cortisol and adrenaline lessen muscle cells' ability to absorb the extra glucose. The body has now been prepared for "fight or flight." Chronic stress will keep blood glucose elevated and may lead to insulin resistance.

Sleep also directly affects blood glucose. Sleep deprivation can impact important hormones involved with glucose metabolism and lead to impaired glucose tolerance, insulin resistance, and dysfunction of the insulin-producing cells of the pancreas.

With our clients, we prioritize both of these important factors in glucose management. In our customized programs, our registered dietitians will work with you to establish realistic stress-reduction practices and healthy sleep routines.

Build Long-Lasting Habits

Following a new dietary pattern for four weeks will jump-start your healing journey, but the secret to continuous improvement and long-term health is building positive habits. Goal-setting and habit-building are foundational in our program. Our mission is to provide you with the education and tools to help you succeed in the long run.

We aspire to help people reverse insulin resistance, place diabetes into remission, and keep it there. If our approach resonates with you and you would like to work with us in a more personalized way, then we hope to see you in one of our programs (visit www.reversingt2d.com)! We'll leave you with our program member Nicole's words:

"When I was diagnosed with type 2 diabetes, it felt like my world caved in around me. My fasting blood glucose was 162 mg/dL; I was scared and didn't know where to begin. Joining your program has changed my life in ways that I can't even begin to describe.

Five weeks into the program and my fasting glucose level went down to 90 mg/dL!! I was back in the non-diabetic range. There aren't enough words in the world to ever adequately express how grateful I am for Diana and Jose, their amazing program, and all the support they give us in the community forum.

They saved my life. The best thing that I did for my health this year, and probably ever, was join their program, and I'll say to anyone wondering whether or not to join, just do it!"

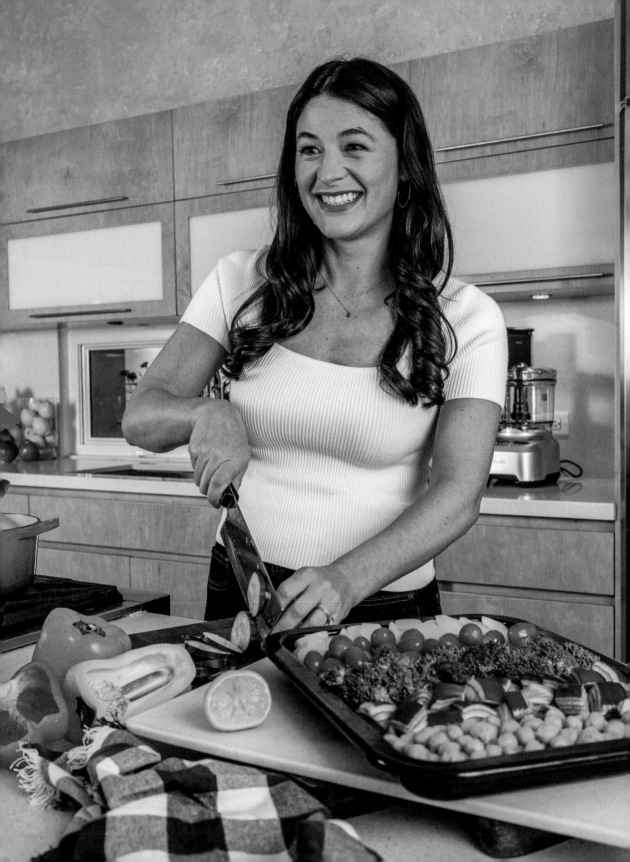

Part 3:
The Recipes

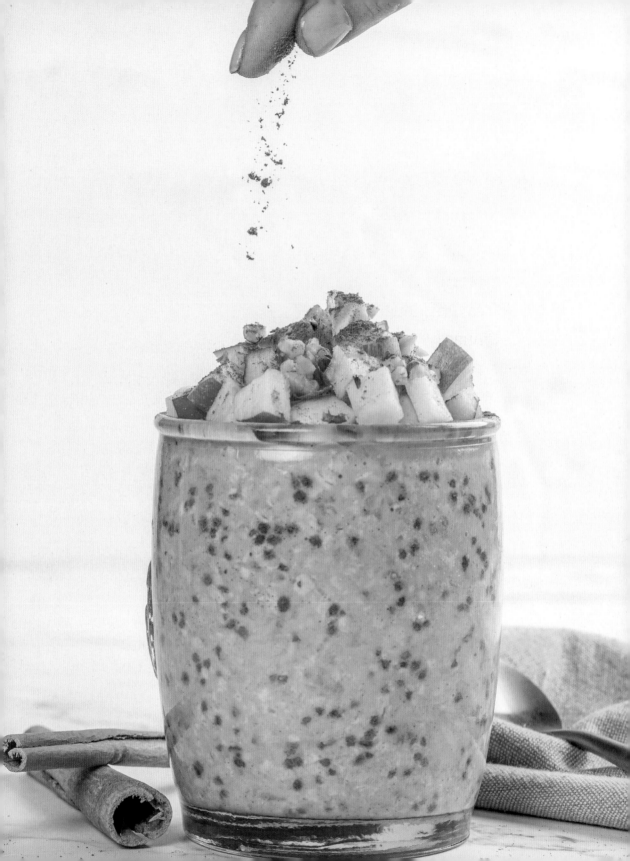

Breakfast

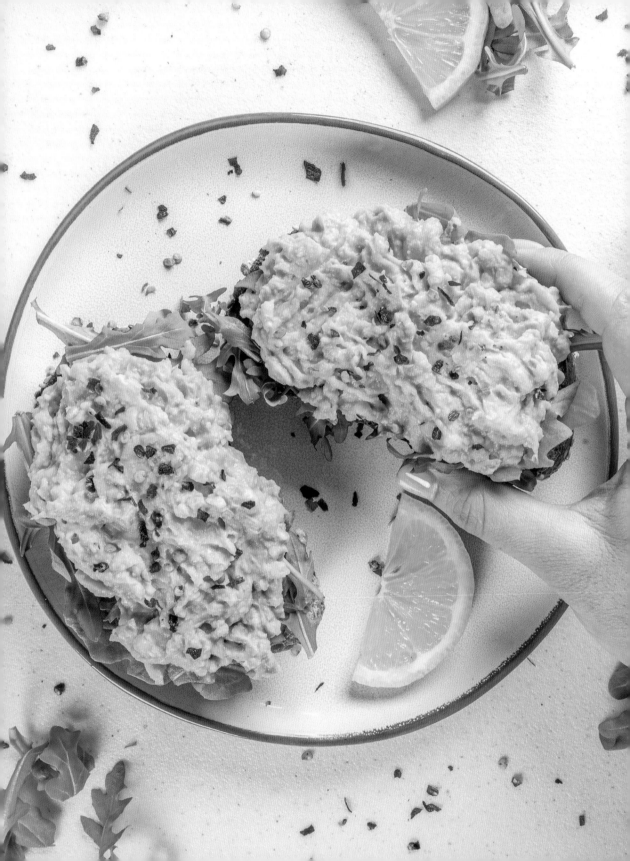

Protein-Packed Avocado Toast

Per Serving: Calories: 434 | Fat: 12g | Carbs: 65g | Fiber: 20g | Protein: 20g

½ cup cooked white beans

¼ medium avocado

1 teaspoon fresh lemon juice

⅛ teaspoon garlic powder

Salt and black pepper, to taste

2 slices whole-grain bread, toasted

1 handful of greens like spinach, kale, or arugula

Red pepper flakes and nutritional yeast, optional

NOTES:

No white beans? Use chickpeas instead.

Add more veggies: Add diced onions and garlic to the avocado-bean mixture. Add tomatoes on top of the toast.

Make it gluten-free: Use gluten-free bread or brown rice cakes.

Serves: 1   🕐 Cooking Time: 10 minutes

Avocado toast has become a culinary icon, but our version packs a secret ingredient—beans! Adding beans to this breakfast staple boosts the protein and fiber content, making it a more balanced meal and more favorable for blood sugar control.

1. In a bowl, mash the white beans, avocado, lemon juice, garlic powder, salt, and pepper together. Continue to mash until you get a guacamole-like consistency.

2. Top the toast with your greens of choice and divide the avocado-bean mixture onto the toast.

3. Sprinkle with the red pepper flakes and nutritional yeast, if desired.

Creamy Chia Seed Pudding

Per Serving: Calories: 405 | Fat: 24g | Carbs: 39g | Fiber: 20g | Protein: 15g

½ cup unsweetened non-dairy yogurt

½ cup unsweetened non-dairy milk

¼ cup chia seeds

1 tablespoon monk fruit sweetener

½ teaspoon vanilla extract

¼ teaspoon ground cinnamon

½ cup fresh berries

Serves: 1   🕐 Cooking Time: 10 minutes, plus 5 hours rest time

Chia seeds are highly nutritious—one 2-tablespoon serving contains almost 10 grams of fiber and countless other nutrients, such as protein, omega-3 fatty acids, and vitamins and minerals including calcium, magnesium, and B vitamins. The high fiber content in this dish helps slow digestion, minimizing blood sugar spikes.

NOTES:

Plan ahead: Make two or more batches and store up to five days in the fridge.

No yogurt? Double the amount of milk.

No monk fruit sweetener? Use a chopped date instead.

Reduce food waste: Use leftover yogurt for the Berry Vanilla Yogurt Parfait (page 115) or Vanilla Latte Smoothie (page 116).

1. Combine all the ingredients, except for the berries, in a jar or sealable container. Let sit for 5 minutes at room temperature.

2. Mix once more to ensure there are no clumps. Place in the fridge for a minimum of 5 hours, or overnight.

3. When ready to eat, top with the berries.

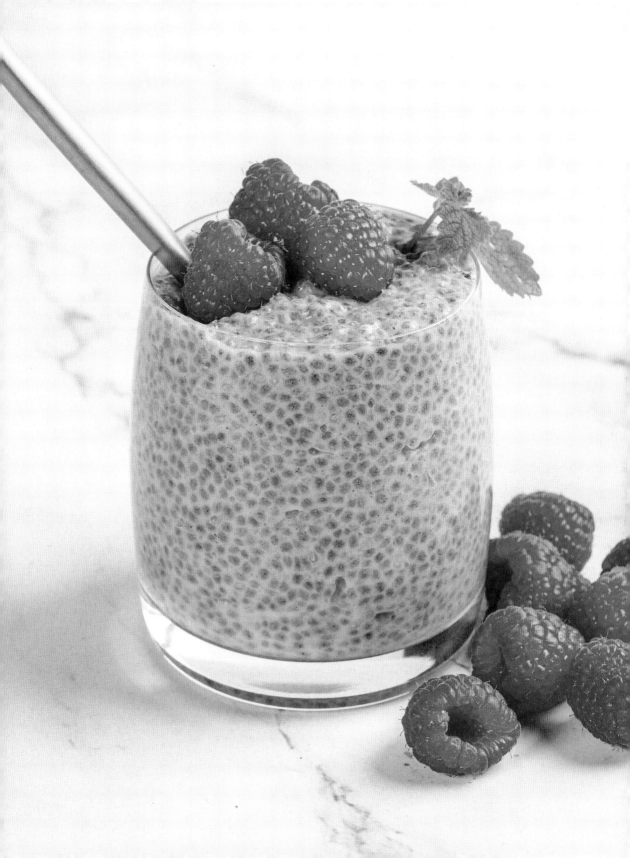

Meal Prep Blueberry Steel-Cut Oats

Per Serving: Calories: 362 | Fat: 11g | Carbs: 52g | Fiber: 12g | Protein: 17g

3 cups unsweetened non-dairy milk

2 cups frozen blueberries

1 cup steel-cut oats

½ cup (about 2 scoops) protein powder, chocolate or vanilla

2 tablespoons ground flaxseed

2 tablespoons chia seeds

2 teaspoons vanilla extract

2 teaspoons ground cinnamon, plus more for serving

Nut butter, optional

NOTES:

Make it gluten-free: Pick gluten-free oats.

Make it nut-free: Use sunflower seed butter for topping.

Serves: 4   🕐 Cooking Time: 25 minutes

Steel-cut oats are a great whole-grain breakfast option. Steel-cut oats have a lower glycemic index than rolled and instant oats, meaning they have less impact on blood sugar. Prep a batch of these blueberry steel-cut oats at the beginning of the week for a hassle-free breakfast.

1. Combine the oats and milk with 3 cups of water in a pot and bring to a boil.

2. Add all the remaining ingredients, except nut butter and fruit, stirring to combine.

3. Reduce the heat to medium-low and simmer for 20–25 minutes, stirring occasionally.

4. Divide the oatmeal into four separate containers and refrigerate until ready to serve.

5. When ready to eat, microwave for 1–2 minutes to reheat. Top with more cinnamon, nut butter, and/or fresh fruit, if desired.

Cinnamon Toasted Muesli

Per ½ cup: Calories: 206 | Fat: 10g | Carbs: 24g | Fiber: 6g | Protein: 7g

3 cups rolled oats

½ cup coconut flakes

⅓ cup ground flaxseed

⅓ cup hemp seeds

⅓ cup chia seeds

⅓ cup pumpkin seeds

½ cup dried raisins

2 teaspoons ground cinnamon

Pinch of salt

NOTES:

Make it gluten-free: Use gluten-free oats.

Use it up: Sprinkle on yogurt, ice cream, Açaí Berry Bowls (page 113), or smoothies, or have a batch in place of cereal topped with fresh fruit.

Serves: 12   🕐 Cooking Time: 20 minutes

Granola is usually high in sugar and low in protein. Our muesli provides a healthier alternative. It's loaded with seeds to give you more fiber, protein, and healthy fats suitable for diabetes. The dried fruit adds a touch of sweetness and more fiber.

1. Preheat the oven to 350°F. Line two baking sheets with parchment paper.

2. Spread the oats on one baking sheet and the coconut flakes, flaxseed, and hemp, chia, and pumpkin seeds on the second.

3. Place the oats on the top rack and the seeds and coconut flakes on the middle rack and bake for 10 minutes, or until lightly toasted in appearance (for crispier oats, broil them on low for an additional 1½ minutes). Once done, let the oats and seeds cool for 5 minutes.

4. Combine the oats, seeds, and all the remaining ingredients in a large bowl and mix thoroughly.

5. Store in a container in a dry pantry for up to one month.

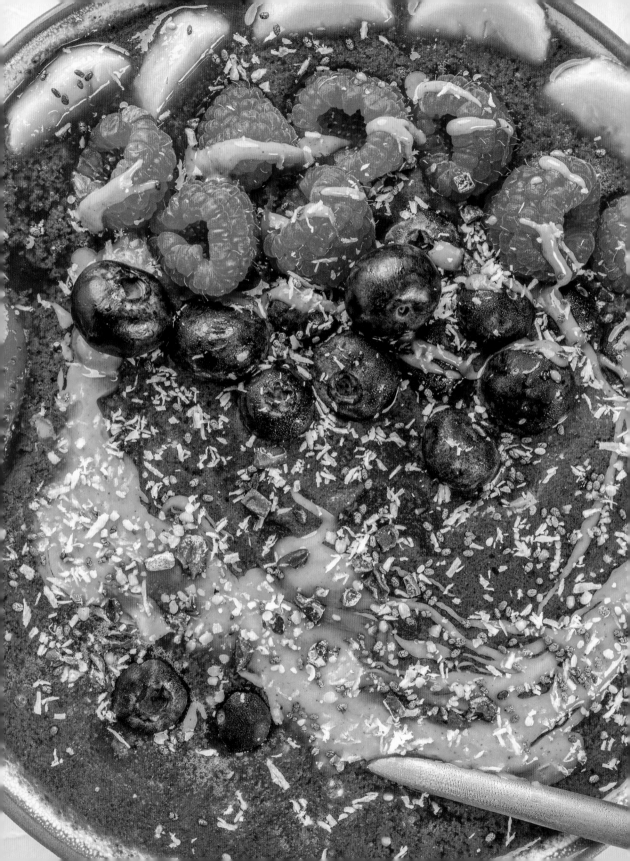

Açaí Berry Bowl

Per bowl: Calories: 418 | Fat: 22g | Carbs: 46g | Fiber: 12g | Protein: 15g

¼ cup unsweetened non-dairy milk

½ cup frozen blueberries

½ cup frozen strawberries

1 (3.5-ounce) packet unsweetened frozen açaí puree

1 tablespoon nut butter

Toppings:

⅓ medium sliced banana

¼ cup berries

1 tablespoon hemp seeds

NOTES:

Shop smart: Frozen açaí puree packets can be found in the freezer section of most grocery stores. Be sure to buy the unsweetened version.

Make it nut-free: Use sunflower seed butter instead of the nut butter.

Add more protein: Add 2 tablespoons (about ½ scoop) of your favorite protein powder.

Add more veggies: Blend in frozen cauliflower rice or zucchini for a creamier texture.

Reduce food waste: Freeze the leftover banana and use it in the No-Sugar-Added Ice Cream (page 202).

Serves: 1   🕐 Cooking Time: 5 minutes

A typical açaí bowl can have anywhere from 21 to 62 grams of added sugar per serving! Our healthier version contains no added sugar and is sweetened only with whole foods. Açaí is packed with antioxidants and fiber, making this bowl excellent for fighting inflammation while also keeping blood sugars balanced.

1. Combine all the ingredients except the toppings in a high-speed blender and puree until completely smooth. Scrape down the sides of the blender as needed to ensure all of the ingredients are evenly blended. When smooth, pour into a bowl.

2. Top with the banana, berries, and hemp seeds.

Tofu Veggie Scramble

Per Serving: Calories: 238 | Fat: 11g | Carbs: 14g | Fiber: 7g | Protein: 27g

¼ cup vegetable stock, plus more as needed

1 red bell pepper, diced

½ yellow onion, diced

1–2 garlic cloves, minced

1 (14-ounce) block tofu, extra firm, drained and pressed

2 tablespoons nutritional yeast

½ teaspoon curry powder

¼ teaspoon salt

Black pepper, to taste

2 handfuls of greens like spinach, kale, or arugula

Whole-grain bread or whole wheat tortillas, optional

NOTES:

Store leftovers: Refrigerate in an airtight container for up to three days.

Add more flavor: Add mushrooms or fresh herbs to the dish.

Make it soy-free: Replace the tofu with a can of chickpeas.

Serves: 2   ◴ Cooking Time: 20 minutes

Tofu is a great plant-based substitute for eggs. Half a cup of tofu has a similar amount of protein as two eggs but with little saturated fat and no cholesterol. Swapping eggs for a tofu scramble doubly benefits blood sugar—the protein contributes to blood sugar regulation and the lack of saturated fat helps improve insulin sensitivity.

1. In a skillet over medium-low heat, combine the vegetable stock with the bell pepper, onion, and garlic. Sauté for 5 minutes, adding more vegetable stock as needed.

2. Break apart the tofu into large chunks and add to the pan. Mash the tofu into smaller pieces using a potato masher or fork right in the pan. Add the nutritional yeast, curry powder, salt, and pepper. Stir to combine the spices evenly and cook for another 7–10 minutes.

3. Add the greens to the pan and stir until just wilted, about 1 minute. Remove the tofu mixture from the heat and adjust the seasonings to taste.

4. Serve with whole-grain bread or in a whole wheat tortilla for a breakfast burrito, if desired.

*Nutrition information is per serving

Berry Vanilla Yogurt Parfait

Per Parfait: Calories: 417 | Fat: 17g | Carbs: 55g | Fiber: 12g | Protein: 16g

½ cup unsweetened non-dairy yogurt

1 tablespoon vanilla protein powder

1 tablespoon peanut or
almond butter

½ teaspoon cinnamon

½ cup berries, fresh or frozen

½ cup whole-grain cereal or
Cinnamon Toasted Muesli
(page 111)

NOTES:

No vanilla protein powder? Use your
flavor of choice.

Make it nut-free: Use sunflower seed
butter in place of the peanut or
almond butter.

Reduce food waste: Use leftover
yogurt in the Creamy Chia Seed
Pudding (page 108) or Vanilla Latte
Smoothie (page 116).

Serves: 1   ○ Cooking Time: 5 minutes

If you're looking for a quick, healthy breakfast option, then look no further. Unlike flavored yogurts, which contain high amounts of added sugar, this parfait contains no-added sugar, helping to keep your blood sugar steady throughout the day.

1. In a small bowl, combine the yogurt, protein powder, peanut butter, and cinnamon. Mix until combined.

2. Add the berries. If using frozen berries, microwave in a microwave-safe bowl for 1 minute. Allow them to cool.

3. Top with the whole-grain cereal or muesli and serve immediately.

Smoothies (4 Ways)

Chocolate Tahini

1 cup unsweetened non-dairy milk

1 frozen ripe banana

1 handful of spinach or baby kale

2 tablespoons cocoa powder

1 tablespoon tahini

Green Machine

1 cup unsweetened non-dairy milk

1 handful of spinach or baby kale

1 stalk celery

½ green apple, cored

½ cup frozen mango

½ cup roughly chopped zucchini

1 tablespoon fresh lemon juice

½ teaspoon grated fresh ginger

Strawberry Banana

1 cup unsweetened non-dairy milk

1 frozen ripe banana

½ cup frozen strawberries

½ cup roughly chopped zucchini

½ teaspoon vanilla extract

Vanilla Latte

1 frozen ripe banana

½ cup unsweetened non-dairy yogurt

½ cup coffee

½ cup roughly chopped zucchini

1–2 tablespoons monk fruit
sweetener or 1–2 Medjool dates

½ teaspoon vanilla extract

Serves: 1   Cooking Time: 5 mins

Smoothies can be a sneaky way to get in more fruit and vegetables. The secret ingredient in many of our smoothies: zucchini! Not only does the zucchini provide a serving of vegetables, it also improves the smoothie's texture.

1. Place all the ingredients in a blender and blend until smooth. Serve immediately.

Per Chocolate Tahini Smoothie:
Calories: 306 | Fat: 14g | Carbs: 41g | Fiber: 10g | Protein: 14g

● Carb-to-Fiber Ratio: 4:1

Per Green Machine Smoothie:
Calories: 210 | Fat: 5g | Carbs: 35g | Fiber: 7g | Protein: 10g

● Carb-to-Fiber Ratio: 5:1

Per Strawberry Banana Smoothie:
Calories: 247 | Fat: 5g | Carbs: 44g | Fiber: 7g | Protein: 10g

● Carb-to-Fiber Ratio: 6:1

Per Vanilla Latte Smoothie:
Calories: 222 | Fat: 7g | Carbs: 36g | Fiber: 6g | Protein: 5g

● Carb-to-Fiber Ratio: 6:1

*Nutrition information is per serving

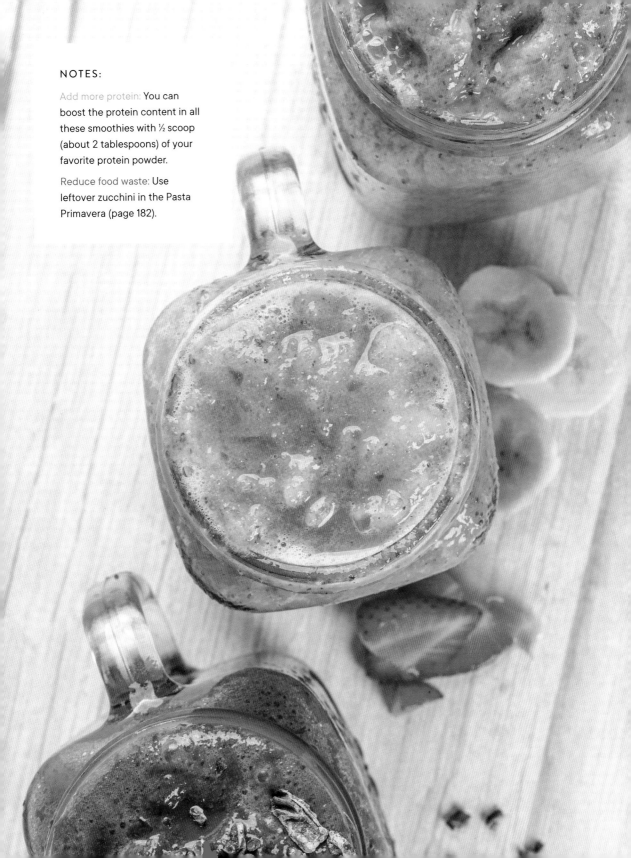

NOTES:

Add more protein: You can boost the protein content in all these smoothies with ½ scoop (about 2 tablespoons) of your favorite protein powder.

Reduce food waste: Use leftover zucchini in the Pasta Primavera (page 182).

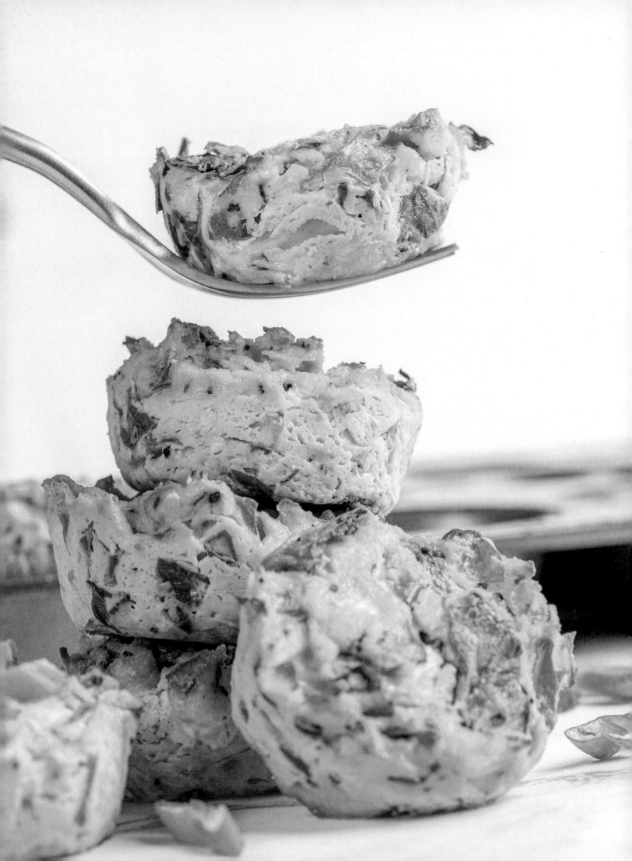

Eggless "Egg" Cups

Per 3 cups: Calories: 163 | Fat: 7g | Carbs: 9g | Fiber: 5g | Protein: 19g

1 (14-ounce) block tofu, extra firm, drained and pressed

½ cup chopped baby spinach

½ bell pepper, finely diced

½ medium yellow onion, finely diced

3 tablespoons nutritional yeast

1 teaspoon ground turmeric

½ teaspoon salt

Black pepper, to taste

Whole-grain bread or fresh fruit, optional

NOTES:

Plan ahead: Make an extra batch of this recipe and store in an airtight container in the fridge for up to five days.

Makes 9 cups   🕐 Cooking Time: 40 minutes

Unlike other egg cup recipes, this version uses tofu to provide protein with little saturated fat. Besides providing coloring similar to eggs, turmeric helps fight inflammation. Turmeric contains curcumin, which is an antioxidant compound with anti-inflammatory properties. The black pepper in this dish helps facilitate its absorption, which is usually quite poor.

1. Preheat the oven to 375°F and prepare a 12-cup muffin tin by spraying it lightly with olive oil cooking spray or lining it with silicone baking cups.

2. Place the tofu in a blender or a food processor and blend until it turns into a paste.

3. Transfer the blended tofu to a bowl and add the rest of the ingredients. Mix well.

4. Pour the mixture into the muffin tin, dividing it evenly among 9 wells.

5. Bake for 25–30 minutes, or until a skewer inserted into the "egg" cups comes out clean.

6. Serve with whole-grain bread and/or fresh fruit, if desired.

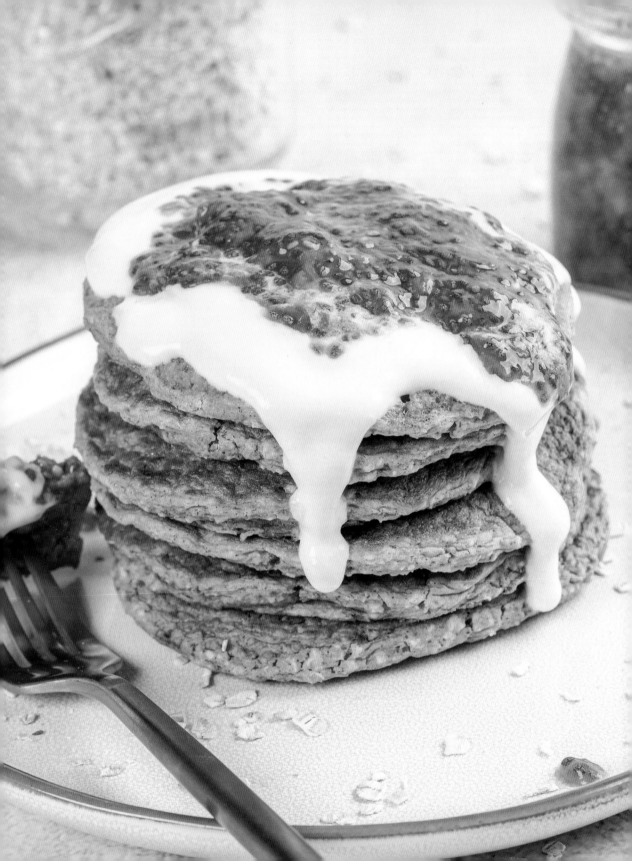

Protein Banana Pancakes

Per 3 pancakes: Calories: 246 | Fat: 5g | Carbs: 38g | Fiber: 6g | Protein: 13g

2 cups rolled oats

2 cups unsweetened non-dairy milk

1 medium ripe banana

¼ cup (about 1 scoop) protein powder, chocolate or vanilla

1 tablespoon baking powder

1 teaspoon ground cinnamon

½ teaspoon salt

OPTIONAL TOPPINGS:

No-Sugar-Added Berry Chia Jam (page 238)

Peanut butter, almond butter, or sunflower seed butter

Fresh fruit

NOTES:

Make it gluten-free: Use gluten-free oats.

Store leftovers: Freeze leftover pancakes for up to three months and pop them in a toaster oven when ready to eat.

Serves: 4   ◷ Cooking Time: 25 minutes

Unlike traditional pancakes, which are usually high in sugar and low in fiber, our version uses bananas for sweetening, rolled oats for fiber, and protein powder for a boost of protein to make this classic breakfast dish suitable for balancing blood sugar levels. Bonus: this recipe is great for when you're unsure of what to do with overripe bananas.

1. Place the oats in a high-speed blender and process until they reach the texture of a flour.

2. Add all the remaining ingredients except the toppings and blend to form a batter. Let the batter sit for 3-5 minutes to thicken.

3. Heat a nonstick pan (or a pan lightly sprayed with oil cooking spray) over medium-low heat. Use a measuring cup to pour in ¼ cup of batter for each pancake.

4. Allow the pancakes to cook until bubbles appear around the edges, 3–5 minutes. Flip and cook on the other side until golden.

5. Add your toppings of choice and serve.

"Ricotta" Toast with Cherry Tomatoes

Per serving: Calories: 325 | Fat: 8g | Carbs: 47g | Fiber: 10g | Protein: 21g

1 cup cherry tomatoes

¼ teaspoon salt

1 serving (½ cup) Herbed "Ricotta" Filling (page 221)

2 slices whole-grain bread, toasted

1 teaspoon balsamic vinegar

Fresh basil or parsley and red pepper flakes, optional

Serves: 1   🕐 Cooking Time: 10 mins

In this recipe, tofu mimics ricotta cheese to provide a high-protein, savory breakfast option. Tofu contains isoflavones (compounds with antioxidant-like properties that can lower inflammation and damage in the body), helping to reduce insulin resistance.

1. Warm a nonstick pan (or a pan lightly sprayed with olive oil cooking spray) over medium heat and add the tomatoes and salt.

2. Sauté the tomatoes until brown, or until soft and skins begin to wrinkle, about 2 minutes.

3. Top each slice of bread with a layer of the tofu "ricotta" filling (about ¼ cup each).

4. Divide the cooked tomatoes on top of the tofu filling and splash with balsamic vinegar.

5. Sprinkle with fresh basil or parsley and red pepper flakes, if desired.

NOTES:

Store leftovers: Refrigerate leftover ricotta filling in an airtight container for up to three days.

Reduce food waste: Use leftover ricotta filling in Eggplant "Ricotta" Roll-Ups (page 175).

Make it gluten-free: Use gluten-free bread instead.

Make it soy-free: Use a cashew-based filling instead of tofu.

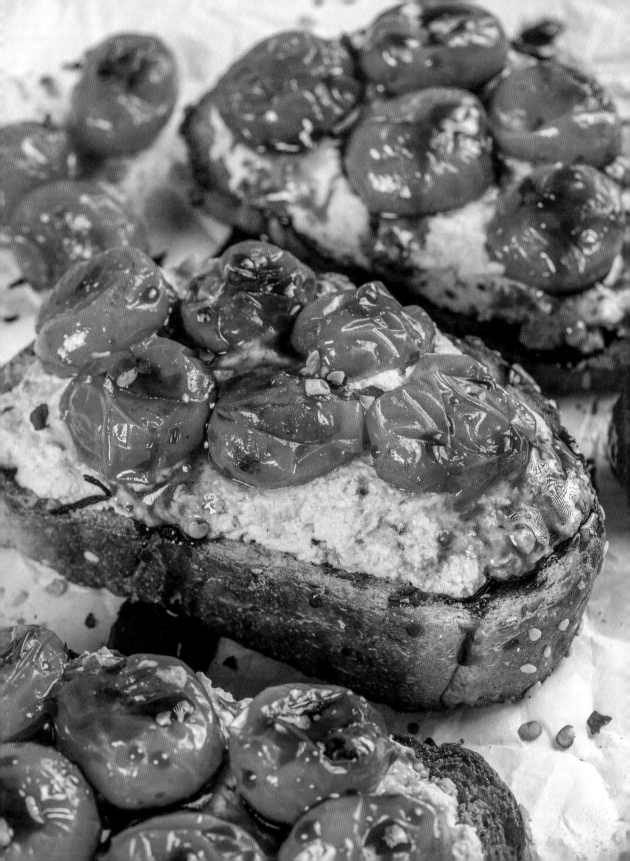

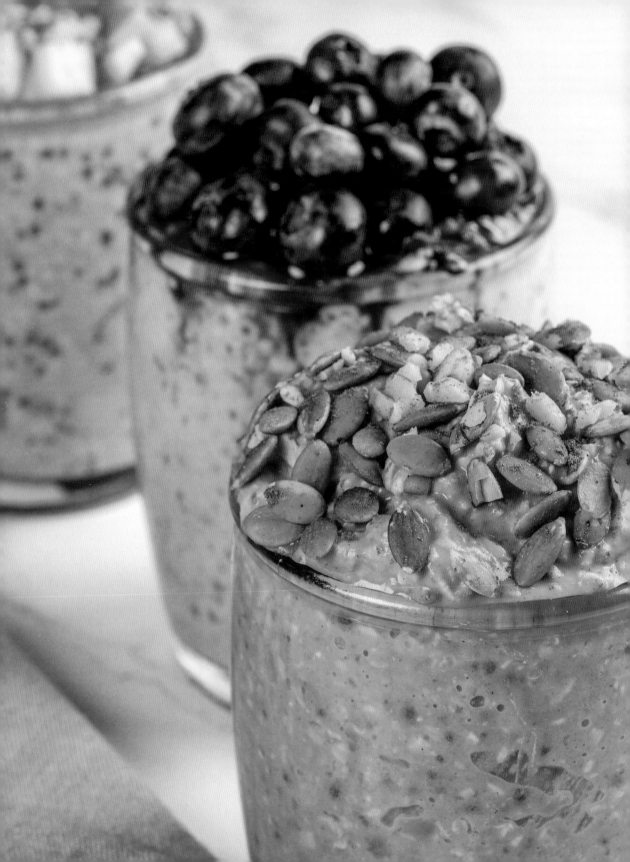

Overnight Oats (3 Ways)

Base Ingredients

¾ cup unsweetened non-dairy milk

½ cup rolled oats

½–1 tablespoon monk fruit sweetener, to taste

2 teaspoons chia seeds

½ teaspoon vanilla extract

Apple Pie

1 apple, finely diced

1 tablespoon crushed walnuts

½ teaspoon ground cinnamon

PB&J

½ cup berries

1 tablespoon peanut butter

Pumpkin Pie

2 tablespoons canned pumpkin

1 tablespoon pepitas

½ teaspoon pumpkin pie spice (or a pinch each of ground nutmeg, cinnamon, and allspice)

NOTES:

Add more protein: Add 2 tablespoons (about ½ scoop) of protein powder.

Make it gluten-free: Use gluten-free oats.

Make it nut-free: Use sunflower seed butter in place of the peanut butter; use sunflower or pumpkin seeds in place of the walnuts.

No monk fruit sweetener? Use a chopped date instead.

Serves: 1   ⏲ Cooking Time: 10 minutes, plus overnight soaking

Overnight oats just take a few minutes to prepare and require no cooking time, making them an excellent weekday breakfast option. These overnight oats contain protein and fiber from rolled oats and chia seeds. Protein and fiber slow digestion, providing a filling and satisfying breakfast that balances blood sugar. Overnight oats are also versatile—they're the perfect vehicle for different spices, fruits, and nuts, keeping your palate excited with every bowl.

1. In a mason jar or glass container, combine all the base ingredients and stir or shake to mix.

2. Add all the ingredients for your variation of choice, then stir or shake to combine.

3. Seal the container and place it in the refrigerator for at least 8 hours, or overnight. When ready to eat, microwave it for 1–2 minutes to reheat. Add a few splashes of milk, if needed, to reach your preferred consistency.

Per Apple Pie jar:
Calories: 384 | Fat: 12g | Carbs: 60g | Fiber: 13g | Protein: 12g

● Carb-to-Fiber Ratio: 5:1

Per PB&J jar:
Calories: 378 | Fat: 16g | Carbs: 48g | Fiber: 11g | Protein: 14g

● Carb-to-Fiber Ratio: 4:1

Per Pumpkin Pie jar:
Calories: 296 | Fat: 11g | Carbs: 37g | Fiber: 9g | Protein: 13g

● Carb-to-Fiber Ratio: 4:1

Blueberry Breakfast Muffins

Per muffin: Calories: 153 | Fat: 3g | Carbs: 27g | Fiber: 5g | Protein: 6g

3 medium ripe bananas

2 cups rolled oats

½ cup unsweetened non-dairy milk

¼ cup (about 1 scoop) protein powder, chocolate or vanilla

2 tablespoons chia seeds

1 tablespoon baking powder

½ teaspoon vanilla extract

Pinch of salt

½ cup blueberries

NOTES:

Change it up: Swap the blueberries for other fruit, or for a dessert muffin, use no-sugar-added chocolate chips.

Make it gluten-free: Use gluten-free oats.

Store leftovers: Freeze leftover muffins for up to three months.

Makes: 8   ◷ Cooking Time: 50 minutes

On average, a store-bought blueberry muffins contain over 400 calories and almost 40 grams (or 10 teaspoons) of added sugar. Our version is made up of health-promoting ingredients including oats, chia seeds, and bananas. Using bananas reduces the muffins' fat and added sugar content, making them more suitable to eat when monitoring blood sugar.

1. Preheat your oven to 350°F. Spray a 12-cup muffin tin with nonstick cooking spray or line it with silicone baking cups.

2. In a high-speed blender or food processor, blend all the ingredients except the blueberries together until combined.

3. Transfer the mixture to a bowl and fold in the blueberries. Pour the mixture into the muffin tin, dividing it evenly among 8 wells. Bake for 35 minutes.

4. Allow the muffins to cool for 10 minutes before serving.

*Nutrition information is per serving

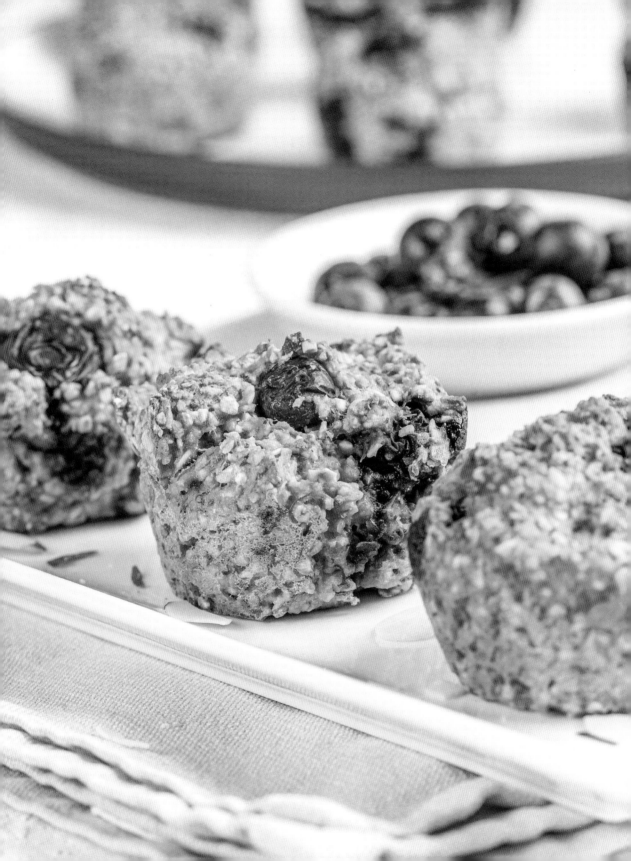

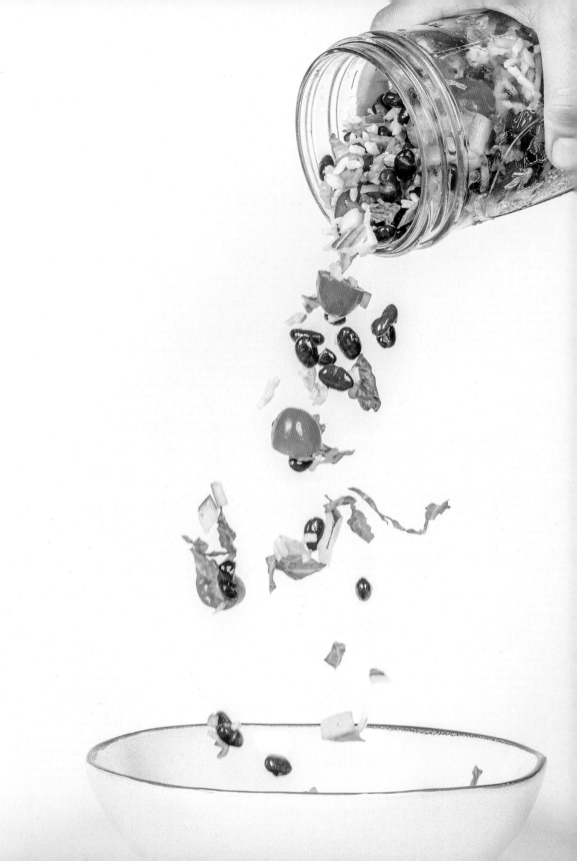

Soups, Sandwiches, and Salads

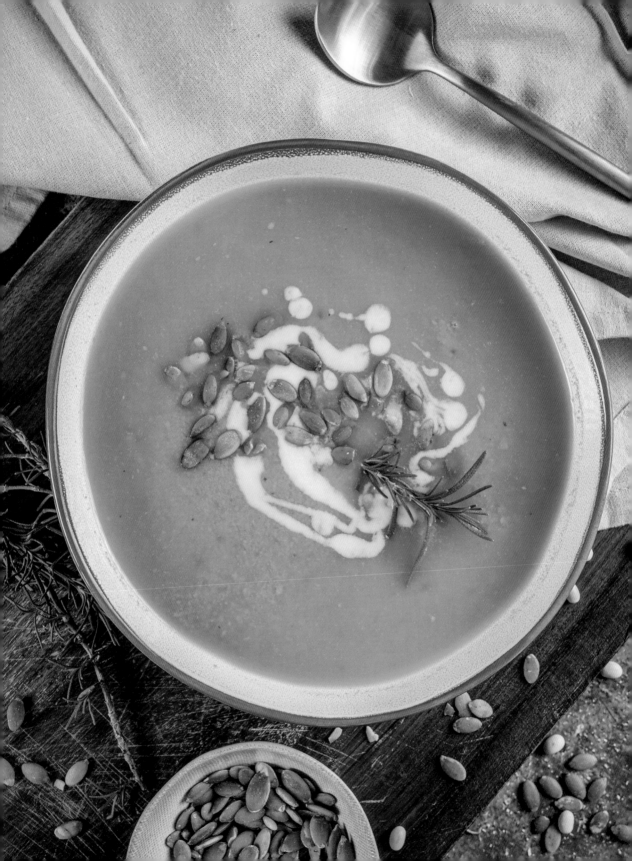

Roasted Pumpkin and White Bean Soup

Per 1⅓ cups: Calories: 237 | Fat: 5g | Carbs: 43g | Fiber: 15g | Protein: 9g

4 cups peeled, cubed pumpkin

1 yellow onion, chopped

4 garlic cloves, chopped

1 tablespoon chopped rosemary

1 (15-ounce) can white beans, drained and rinsed

1 ½ cups vegetable stock, plus more for sautéing

1 cup light canned coconut milk

½ teaspoon salt, or more to taste

¼ teaspoon black pepper

NOTES:

Store leftovers: Freeze in a freezer bag or airtight container for one to two months.

Revise accordingly: Depending on the vegetable stock you use (i.e. low-sodium vs. regular), you may have to adjust the salt quantity.

Serves: 4   🕐 Cooking Time: 1 hour

Pumpkin gets its bright-orange color from an antioxidant called beta-carotene. In the body, beta-carotene turns into vitamin A, which is important for healthy vision, to fight infections, and for maintaining healthy skin. We added white beans to this soup to pack it with protein for a filling, balanced meal.

1. Preheat oven to 350°F and line a baking sheet with parchment paper.

2. Bake the pumpkin for 20–25 minutes, or until fork-tender.

3. Meanwhile, in a stockpot over medium heat, sauté the onions, garlic, and rosemary in a splash of vegetable stock. Cook until the onions become translucent, 2 to 3 minutes, adding more vegetable stock as needed.

4. Add the pumpkin and white beans to the pot, stirring to combine. Cook for about 2 minutes.

5. Add the vegetable stock and bring to a boil, then reduce heat and simmer for about 25 minutes.

6. Stir in the coconut milk, salt, and pepper.

7. Using an immersion blender or working in batches in a blender, blend the soup until creamy. Serve immediately.

*Nutrition information is per serving

Chickpea Noodle Soup

Per 1½ cups: Calories: 226 | Fat: 3g | Carbs: 42g | Fiber: 10g | Protein: 10g

1 medium yellow onion, diced

4 garlic cloves, minced

2 medium carrots, diced

3 stalks celery, diced

2 bay leaves

3 sprigs fresh thyme or ½ teaspoon dried thyme

8 cups vegetable stock, plus more for sautéing

2 (15-ounce) cans chickpeas, drained and rinsed

3 ounces (2 cups) whole-wheat pasta or noodles

2 cups chopped kale

1 teaspoon salt, or more to taste

½ teaspoon black pepper, or to taste

Juice of ½ large lemon

¼ cup finely chopped fresh parsley

NOTES:

Make it gluten-free: Use quinoa, rice, or lentil pasta.

Reduce food waste: Use leftover ingredients to make the White Bean and Lemon Kale Soup (page 137).

Revise accordingly: Depending on the vegetable stock you use (i.e. low-sodium vs. regular), you may have to adjust the salt quantity.

Serves: 6   ⏱ Cooking Time: 40 minutes

Like a minestrone, this chickpea and noodle dish packs in the fiber with seasonal vegetables, kale, whole-grain pasta, and chickpeas for a diabetes-friendly comforting soup. For even more blood sugar control, cook the noodles al dente to lower their glycemic index.

1. In a stockpot, sauté the onion and garlic in a few splashes of vegetable stock over low heat for 2 to 3 minutes, stirring frequently, adding more vegetable stock as needed to prevent the onions from browning.

2. Add the carrots and celery and cook for another 7 to 10 minutes, or until carrots are soft, adding more vegetable stock as needed.

3. Add the bay leaves, thyme, vegetable stock, and chickpeas and bring to a low simmer.

4. Cook for about 20 minutes at a low simmer, partially covered.

5. Stir the noodles into the soup and cook until done, 6–10 minutes depending on the type of noodles used. Add more water or stock as needed, if too much liquid evaporates.

6. Toss in the kale, salt, and pepper and stir until the kale is gently wilted.

7. Stir in the lemon juice and parsley and serve.

*Nutrition information is per serving

Tofu Bok Choy Noodle Soup

Per 2 cups: Calories: 197 | Fat: 5g | Carbs: 27g | Fiber: 4g | Protein: 14g

4 garlic cloves, minced

¼ cup minced fresh ginger

1 bunch green onions, chopped and divided into green and white parts

6 cups vegetable stock, plus more for sautéing

1 large head bok choy, chopped and divided into stems and leaves (about 4 cups)

2 cups mushrooms of choice

1 (14-ounce) block tofu, firm, cut into ½-inch cubes

4 ounces brown rice noodles

6 tablespoons less-sodium soy sauce or tamari

¼ teaspoon red pepper flakes, optional

NOTES:

Make it soy-free: Omit the tofu or replace it with seitan. Use coconut aminos in place of the soy sauce.

Revise accordingly: Depending on the vegetable stock you use (i.e. low-sodium vs. regular), you may have to adjust the soy sauce quantity.

Serves: 5   ◷ Cooking Time: 25 minutes

This tofu bok choy noodle soup is comforting and aromatic. Besides adding flavor and spice, ginger may reduce blood sugar levels. Opting for whole-grain noodles increases the fiber content and makes this dish even more blood sugar-friendly.

1. In a stockpot over medium-low heat, sauté the garlic, ginger, and the white parts of the green onions in a few splashes of vegetable stock. Cook, stirring occasionally, for 2–3 minutes.

2. Pour in the vegetable stock and 3 cups of water. Bring to a boil, then reduce to a simmer and cook for 5 minutes.

3. Add the bok choy stems to the pot and cook for 5 minutes, or until the stems start to become tender.

4. Add the bok choy leaves, mushrooms, tofu, and noodles to the pot and cook for another 5 minutes, until the leaves and mushrooms are tender and the noodles are cooked.

5. Stir in the soy sauce and the red pepper flakes, if using.

6. Serve topped with the green parts of the green onion.

Hearty 3-Bean Chili

Per 1¼ cups: Calories: 285 | Fat: 3g | Carbs: 58g | Fiber: 23g | Protein: 18g

1 yellow onion, diced

1 bell pepper, diced

3 garlic cloves, minced

1 jalapeño, seeded and diced

2 cups vegetable stock, plus more for sautéing

2 (14.5-ounce) cans diced tomatoes

1 (15-ounce) can black beans, drained and rinsed

1 (15-ounce) can pinto beans, drained and rinsed

1 (15-ounce) can chickpeas, drained and rinsed

1 cup corn, frozen or canned

1 cup riced cauliflower, frozen or fresh

1 tablespoon tomato paste

1 tablespoon chili powder

½ teaspoon ground cumin

½ teaspoon dried oregano

½ teaspoon garlic powder

½ teaspoon onion powder

½ teaspoon paprika

1 teaspoon salt, or more to taste

½ teaspoon red pepper flakes

¼ teaspoon black pepper

OPTIONAL TOPPINGS:

Sliced avocado

Cashew Sour Cream (page 241)

Serves: 6   🕐 Cooking Time: 30 minutes

Beans are a plant-based powerhouse due to their high fiber and protein content. And this chili has three types of beans! What's more, having beans as your source of protein can help improve blood sugar control and insulin sensitivity.

1. Place a splash of vegetable stock in a pressure cooker and set the cooker to sauté. Add the onion, bell pepper, garlic, and jalapeño and sauté for 3 minutes, adding more stock as needed to prevent the vegetables from sticking.

2. Turn off the heat and add all the remaining ingredients except the toppings. Stir to combine.

3. Close the pressure cooker, lock the lid, and pressure cook on high for 15 minutes.

4. Allow the pressure to naturally release for 10 minutes, then manually release any remaining pressure.

5. Serve with your toppings of choice.

*Nutrition information is per serving

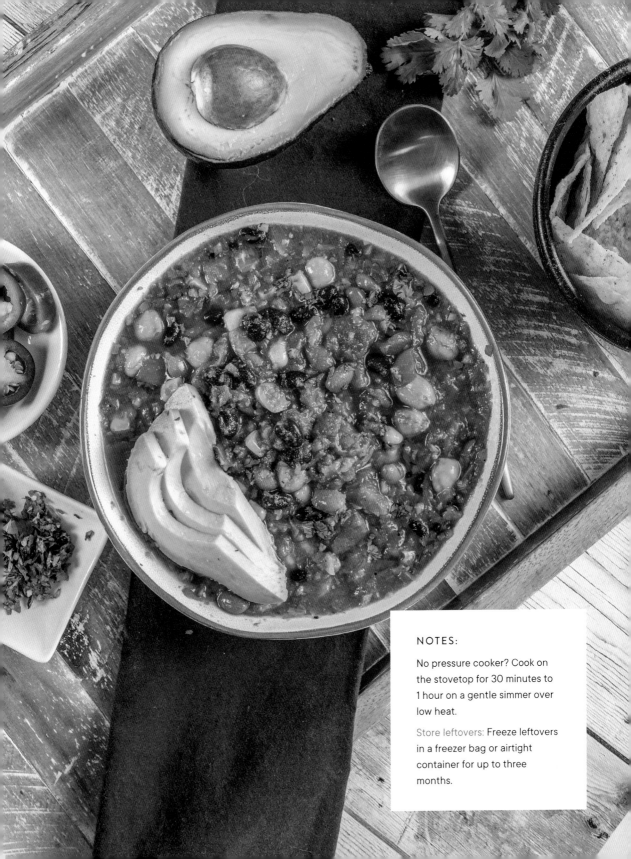

NOTES:

No pressure cooker? Cook on the stovetop for 30 minutes to 1 hour on a gentle simmer over low heat.

Store leftovers: Freeze leftovers in a freezer bag or airtight container for up to three months.

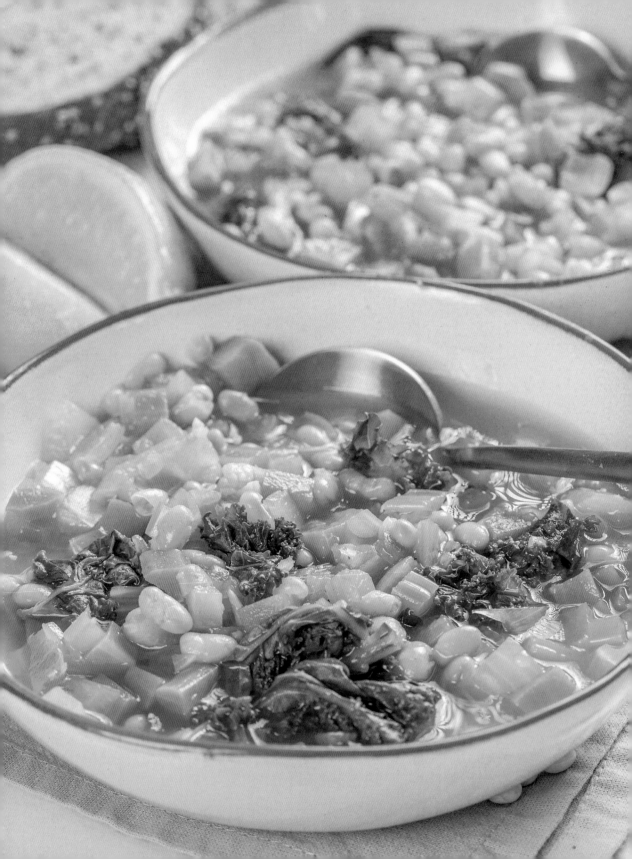

White Bean and Lemon Kale Soup

Per 1½ cups: Calories: 203 | Fat: 1g | Carbs: 39g | Fiber: 11g | Protein: 9g

1 large yellow onion, chopped

3 garlic cloves, minced

2 medium carrots, chopped

2 celery stalks, chopped

6 cups vegetable stock, plus more
for sautéing

3 (15-ounce) cans cannellini beans,
drained and rinsed

2 teaspoons dried oregano

2 teaspoons dried thyme

3–4 cups chopped kale leaves,
stems removed

¼ cup fresh lemon juice

½ teaspoon salt, or more to taste

½ teaspoon black pepper

⅓ cup fresh parsley, chopped

Serves: 6   🕐 **Cooking Time: 30 minutes**

This white bean and lemon kale soup is packed with nutrients beneficial for blood sugar. The white beans and kale provide loads of fiber to slow digestion and regulate blood sugar, while the parsley and lemon juice contribute vitamin C and antioxidants to help fight damage caused by insulin resistance.

1. In a stockpot, sauté the onion and garlic in a few splashes of vegetable stock over low heat for 2 to 3 minutes, stirring frequently, adding more vegetable stock as needed to prevent the onions from browning.

2. Add the carrots and celery and cook for another 7 to 10 minutes, or until carrots are soft, adding more vegetable stock as needed.

3. Add the vegetable stock, beans, oregano, and thyme, and stir.

4. Bring to a boil, then reduce the heat to medium-low and let simmer over medium-low heat for 15 minutes, uncovered.

5. Add the kale, stir, and continue cooking for 3–4 minutes, until the kale is wilted.

6. Blend 1–2 cups of the soup in a blender or using an immersion blender, then return it to the pot.

7. Add the lemon juice, salt, and pepper, and top with the parsley before serving.

NOTES:

Store leftovers: Freeze in a freezer bag or airtight container for up to three months.

Add additional toppings: Top with red pepper flakes and/or nutritional yeast.

Reduce food waste: Use leftover ingredients to make the Chickpea Noodle Soup (page 132).

Revise accordingly: Depending on the vegetable stock you use (i.e. low-sodium vs. regular), you may have to adjust the salt quantity.

*Nutrition information is per serving

Classic Lentil Soup

Per 1 cup: Calories: 208 | Fat: 1g | Carbs: 39g | Fiber: 7g | Protein: 14g

½ medium yellow onion, diced

2 garlic cloves, minced

½ large carrot, chopped

1 celery rib, chopped

1 cup dried brown lentils, rinsed

½ (14-ounce) can fire-roasted crushed tomatoes

3 cups vegetable stock, plus more for sautéing

½ teaspoon paprika

¼ teaspoon cumin

¼ teaspoon chili powder

1 dried bay leaf

2 cups spinach

1 tablespoon lemon juice

¼ teaspoon salt, or more to taste

¼ teaspoon pepper

Serves: 4   🕐 Cooking Time: 30 minutes

Lentils are a plant-based powerhouse, serving 18 grams of protein and 16 grams of fiber per cup. This lentil soup is thick and creamy and incorporates spinach for even more fiber to help maintain blood sugar levels.

1. In a stockpot, sauté the onion and garlic in a few splashes of vegetable stock over low heat for 2 to 3 minutes, stirring frequently, adding more vegetable stock as needed to prevent the onions from browning.

2. Add the carrots and celery and cook for another 7 to 10 minutes, or until carrots are soft, adding more vegetable stock as needed.

3. Add the vegetable stock, paprika, cumin, chili powder, and bay leaf. Stir.

4. Increase the heat and bring to a simmer. Cover and turn heat down to medium-low. Simmer for 35 to 40 minutes, or until lentils are soft.

5. To thicken the soup, remove the bay leaf and transfer 1 cup to a blender, and blend until creamy, then transfer it back into the pot.

6. Add the spinach and cook for another 1 to 2 minutes, or until the spinach is wilted.

7. Add lemon juice, salt, and pepper. To adjust the soup's consistency add a touch more vegetable stock, if desired.

NOTES:

Store leftovers: Refrigerate in an airtight container for three to five days or freeze for up to three months.

Revise accordingly: Depending on the vegetable stock you use (i.e. low-sodium vs. regular), you may have to adjust the salt quantity.

*Nutrition information is per serving

Chickpea Toona Lettuce Wraps

Per serving: Calories: 355 | Fat:18g | Carbs: 39g | Fiber: 12g | Protein: 12g

1 (15-ounce) can chickpeas, drained and rinsed

1 celery stalk, chopped

3 tablespoons Eggless Mayo (page 240) or store-bought vegan mayo

2 tablespoons minced onion, white or red

1 tablespoon capers, chopped

½ teaspoon caper brine

¼ teaspoon salt

¼ teaspoon black pepper

Romaine lettuce leaves

Serves: 2   ⏱ Cooking Time: 10 minutes

This chickpea toona salad brings the flavor of a traditional tuna salad without the fish. Capers add saltiness to the dish, while our Eggless Mayo keeps the salad free of saturated fat.

1. In a bowl, mash the chickpeas with the back of a fork, leaving a few whole chickpeas.

2. Add all the remaining ingredients except the romaine leaves and stir to combine.

3. Serve in romaine lettuce wraps.

NOTES:

No romaine? Use Boston bibb lettuce, collard greens, or cabbage leaves.

No chickpeas? Use white beans instead.

Store leftovers: Refrigerate the leftover chickpea mix in a sealed container for up to two days.

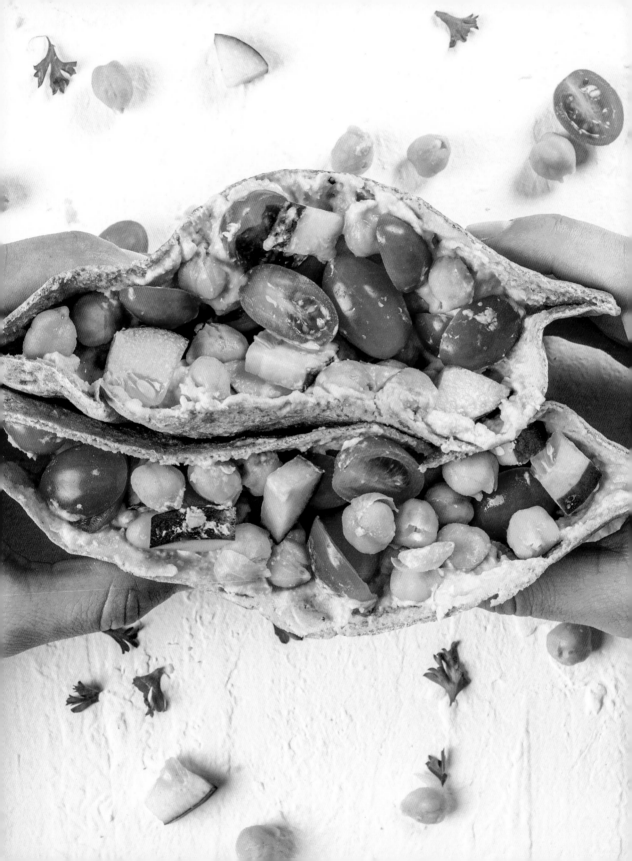

Chopped Salad Pita Pockets

Per pita: Calories: 403 | Fat: 9g | Carbs: 70g | Fiber: 13g | Protein: 17g

½ cup cooked chickpeas

½ cup diced cucumber

¼ cup sliced cherry tomatoes

¼ teaspoon salt, plus more to taste

2 tablespoons Oil-Free Hummus (page 226) or store-bought hummus

1 whole-wheat pita, halved, or 2 mini whole-wheat pitas

Serves: 1   ◷ Cooking Time: 10 minutes

Cucumbers have a low glycemic index of 15, which makes them a highly favorable vegetable for blood sugar. Due to their low glycemic index, adding cucumbers to a dish can bulk it up without significantly impacting blood sugar. These chopped salad pita pockets pair cucumbers with whole-wheat pitas, chickpeas, and additional vegetables to create a simple but filling meal.

NOTES:

Make it gluten-free: Use lettuce wraps, collard greens, brown rice tortillas, or gluten-free flatbread instead of the pita.

Add more flavor: Add lime juice, fresh herbs, or spices to the chickpea mixture.

Add additional toppings: Add bell peppers, red onions, and/or black olives.

No chickpeas? Use marinated tofu, white beans, or lentils instead.

1. In a bowl, combine the chickpeas, cucumber, tomatoes, and salt. Adjust the salt as needed.

2. Gently open each pita half to create a pocket. Evenly spread a thin layer of the hummus inside each pita pocket.

3. Stuff the pita pockets with the chickpea mixture and serve.

Creamy Chickpea Avocado Sandwich

Per sandwich: Calories: 446 | Fat: 13g | Carbs: 65g | Fiber: 17g | Protein: 21g

½ cup cooked chickpeas

¼ medium avocado

1 teaspoon fresh lemon juice

¼ teaspoon salt

Black pepper, to taste

2 slices whole-grain bread, toasted

2–3 slices tomato

1 handful of greens, such as arugula, spinach, or romaine

Serves: 1   🕐 Cooking Time: 10

Use chickpeas as a sandwich filling to create a fiber- and protein-packed lunch favorable for blood sugar. The whole-grain bread and vegetables in this recipe add even more fiber and protein, so you stay full and maintain balanced blood sugar throughout the afternoon.

1. In a large bowl, combine the chickpeas and avocado. Mash well until everything is combined. Add the lemon juice, salt, and pepper. Mix well once more.

2. Top one slice of the toast with the greens and tomatoes. Add the mashed chickpea mixture and top with the other slice of toast.

NOTES:

Add more flavor: Add garlic or fresh herbs, such as dill or parsley, to the chickpea mixture.

Make it gluten-free: Use gluten-free bread, brown rice tortillas, or lettuce wraps.

Store leftovers: Refrigerate the leftover chickpea-avocado mix in a sealed container for up to two days.

*Nutrition information is per serving

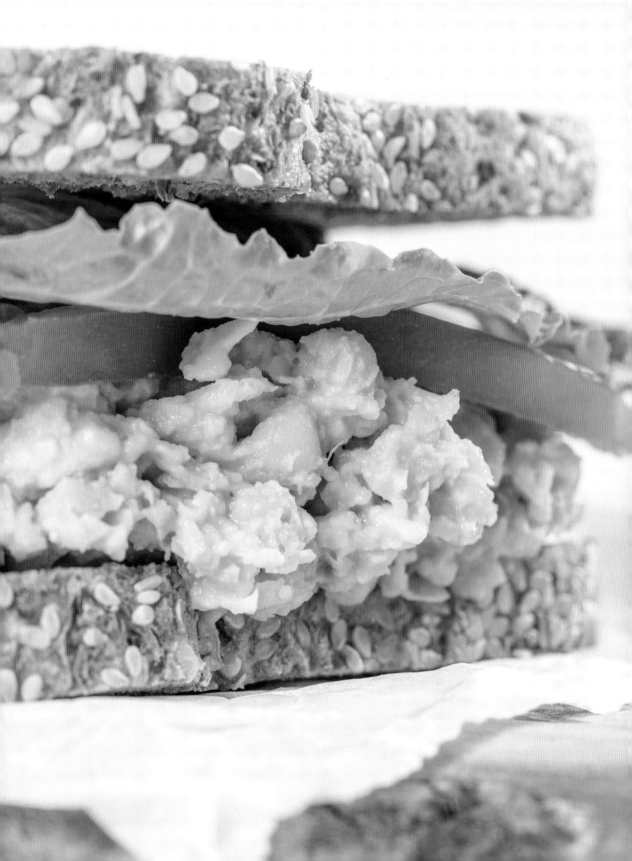

Tempeh, Lettuce, and Tomato Sandwich

Per sandwich: Calories: 539 | Fat: 22g | Carbs: 53g | Fiber: 10g | Protein: 36g

2 tablespoons less-sodium soy sauce, tamari, or coconut aminos

1 tablespoon vegetable stock

2 teaspoons balsamic vinegar

½ teaspoon chili powder

¼ teaspoon paprika

Salt and black pepper, to taste

3 ½ ounces tempeh (about ⅓ of a package), cut into slices

2 teaspoons Eggless Mayo (page 240) or store-bought vegan mayonnaise

1 teaspoon Dijon or yellow mustard

2 slices whole-grain bread, toasted

Romaine lettuce leaves

½ small tomato, sliced

Serves: 1   🕐 Cooking Time: 40 mins

Tempeh is a high-protein, plant-based food made from fermented soybeans. The texture is dry and firm, with a slightly nutty taste. In this recipe, tempeh soaks up the marinade flavors to provide a plant-based alternative to the classic BLT that's much lower in saturated fat.

1. Preheat the oven to 375°F. Line a baking sheet with parchment paper.

2. In a zipper-lock bag or shallow bowl, mix the soy sauce, vegetable stock, balsamic vinegar, chili powder, paprika, salt, and pepper together. Add the tempeh and let it marinate for 10–15 minutes.

3. Arrange the tempeh in an even layer on the baking sheet. Bake for 18–20 minutes, flipping halfway through. Remove from the oven and set aside.

4. Spread the mayo and mustard on one slice of toast. Layer the romaine, tomato, and tempeh on the toast, and season to taste with salt and pepper. Close the sandwich and enjoy!

NOTES:

Store leftovers: This is best assembled just before serving. The tempeh can be prepared and cooked in advance and kept in the fridge for up to four days.

*Nutrition information is per serving

Roasted Sweet Potato Salad with Arugula and Millet

Per 1 cup: Calories: 375 | Fat: 16g | Carbs: 48g | Fiber: 9g | Protein: 12g

3 cups peeled, cubed sweet potato (2–3 potatoes)

½ teaspoon salt, plus more to taste

1 yellow onion, thinly sliced

½ cup millet

1 (15-ounce can) chickpeas, drained and rinsed

3 cups arugula

½ cup walnuts, chopped

½ batch Creamy Balsamic Vinaigrette (page 244)

Black pepper, to taste

NOTES:

Add more veggies: Add more arugula to increase the volume of the serving without significantly changing the nutritional profile.

Store leftovers: Divide the salad into airtight containers and store in the refrigerator for up to four days. Add the dressing just before serving.

Save time: Cook the millet in an Instant Pot® or other electric multi-cooker.

Serves: 5   Cooking Time: 45 minutes

Millet is an ancient grain that is naturally gluten-free and high in protein and fiber. Regular consumption of millet has been shown to reduce blood sugar levels and improve insulin resistance.

1. Preheat the oven to 425°F. Line a large baking sheet with parchment paper.

2. Spread the cubed sweet potatoes on the baking sheet in an even layer. Spray with olive oil cooking spray, add the salt, and toss to coat. Bake for 15 minutes, then add the sliced onions and return to the oven for another 15 minutes. Remove from the oven and set aside.

3. Meanwhile, combine the millet and 1 cup water in a saucepan. Bring the water to a boil, then decrease the heat to low and cover. Allow the millet to simmer for about 15 minutes, stir, then remove from the heat and allow to sit, covered, for an additional 10 minutes.

4. Once the millet has fully absorbed the water, fluff it with a fork and transfer it to a large bowl. Add the roasted sweet potatoes and onions, chickpeas, arugula, and walnuts.

5. When ready to serve, add the dressing and toss until well combined.

6. Add salt and pepper to taste and serve.

Black Bean and Corn Salad

Per 1½ cups: Calories: 365 | Fat: 12g | Carbs: 55g | Fiber: 19g | Protein: 17g

½ cup diced white onions

2 tablespoons apple cider vinegar

1 ¼ teaspoons salt, divided

2 tablespoons fresh lime juice

2 garlic cloves, minced

2 (15-ounce) cans black beans, drained and rinsed

1 ½ cups corn, frozen or canned

3 plum tomatoes, chopped

½ cup chopped fresh cilantro

½ teaspoon black pepper

½ batch (½ cup) Green Goddess Drizzle (page 243), optional

NOTES:

Change it up: Serve in lettuce wraps, or with quinoa or brown rice.

Serves: 4-6   🕐 Cooking Time: 20 minutes

Sweet corn has a low glycemic index and is full of fiber and other nutrients. Pairing corn with black beans creates a protein- and fiber-dense salad that's great for regulating blood sugar.

1. In a small bowl, combine the onions, apple cider vinegar, ¼ teaspoon of the salt, and 3 tablespoons of water. Set aside to marinate.

2. Meanwhile, in a large bowl, whisk together the lime juice, garlic, and the remaining 1 teaspoon of salt.

3. Add the beans, corn, tomatoes, cilantro, and pepper to the bowl and mix until the vegetables and beans are evenly coated with the lime juice.

4. Drain the onions and add to the bowl. Toss one last time until combined.

5. When ready to serve, add the dressing, if desired, and toss.

*Nutrition information is per serving

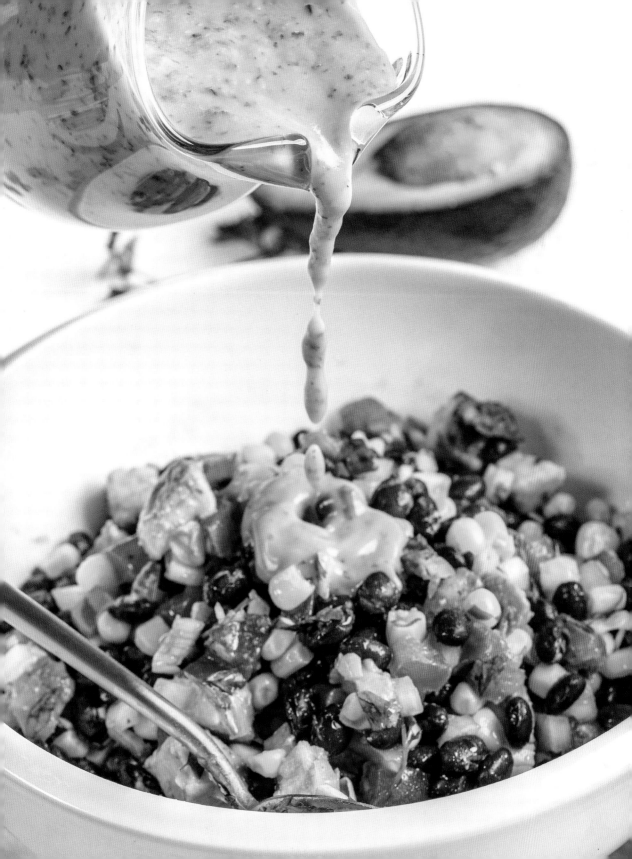

Crunchy Salad with Peanut Dressing

Per 1½ cups: Calories: 316 | Fat: 21g | Carbs: 20g | Fiber: 6g | Protein: 20g

1 (14-ounce) block tofu, extra firm, drained and pressed

½ teaspoon garlic powder

½ teaspoon onion powder

1 cucumber, seeded and cut into matchsticks

1 red bell pepper, cut into matchsticks

2 cups chopped purple cabbage

2 large carrots, peeled and shredded

3 cups chopped romaine lettuce

2 tablespoons chopped fresh cilantro

½ cup roasted peanuts, chopped

Dressing

¼ small red onion, thinly sliced

3 garlic cloves, minced

1 tablespoon grated fresh ginger

1–2 teaspoons monk fruit sweetener

3 tablespoons rice vinegar

3 tablespoons peanut butter

2 teaspoons fresh lime juice

1 ½ tablespoons less-sodium soy sauce or tamari

Serves: 4   🕐 Cooking Time: 40 minutes

Staying hydrated can help keep blood sugar levels in check. The vegetables in this crunchy salad have a high water content, contributing to your daily fluid needs and aiding blood sugar management.

1. Preheat the oven to 400°F. Line a baking sheet with parchment paper.

2. Once the oven is preheated, dice the tofu into ¼-inch cubes and toss them with the garlic and onion powder. Spread onto the prepared baking sheet and bake for 25 minutes, or until the tofu is crisp and firm to the touch.

3. Combine all the dressing ingredients plus 1 tablespoon of water in a bowl and whisk until fully combined.

4. Mix the cucumber, bell pepper, cabbage, carrots, lettuce, tofu, and dressing together in a large bowl until well combined.

5. Garnish with the cilantro and peanuts and serve.

NOTES:

Save time: Buy precut veggies.

Make it soy-free: Swap the tofu for your choice of beans. Use coconut aminos in place of the soy sauce.

*Nutrition information is per serving

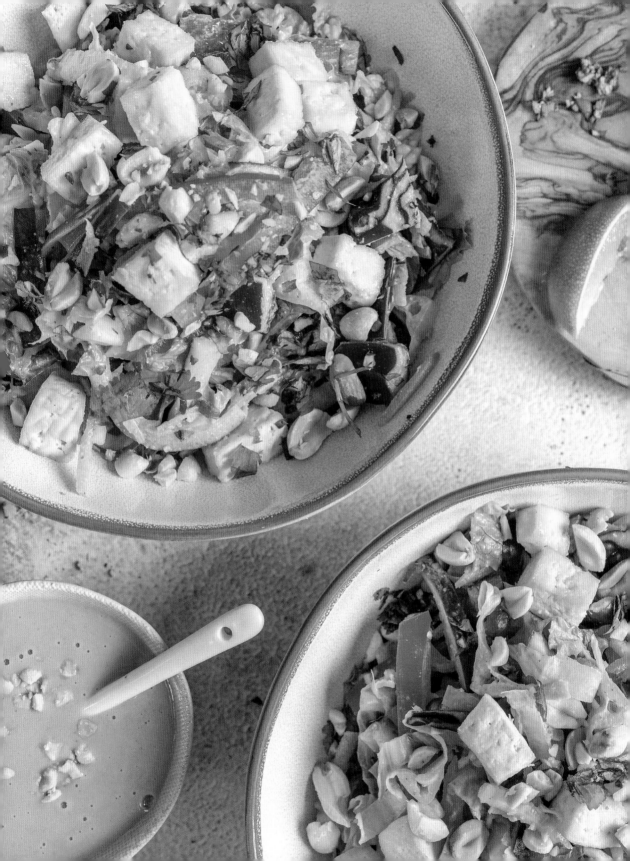

Black Bean Farro Salad

Per 1¼ cups: Calories: 270 | Fat: 2g | Carbs: 51g | Fiber: 9g | Protein: 13g

1 cup farro

1 (15-ounce) can black beans, drained and rinsed

½ red bell pepper, chopped

½ carrot, grated

¼ cup chopped fresh parsley

3 green onions, chopped

2 garlic cloves, minced

2 tablespoons fresh lemon juice

1 teaspoon salt

½ tablespoon olive oil, optional

Serves: 4   🕐 Cooking Time: 35 minutes

Farro is a very nutritious ancient grain that works well as a salad base. It's an excellent source of protein, fiber, and minerals like magnesium and zinc, all important nutrients for blood sugar regulation.

1. Prepare the farro according to the package instructions.

2. Transfer the cooked farro to a large bowl, add all the remaining ingredients, and mix until everything is well combined.

NOTES:

Make it gluten-free: Use quinoa, brown rice, or millet in place of the farro.

Save time: Cook the farro in an Instant Pot® or other electric multi-cooker.

*Nutrition information is per serving

Simple Green Salad

Per serving (without dressing): Calories: 65 | Fat: 1g | Carbs: 13g | Fiber: 4g | Protein: 4g

3 cups (loosely packed) mixed greens or lettuce of choice, torn into bite-size pieces

½ small cucumber, chopped

½ cup sliced cherry tomatoes

¼ small red onion, thinly sliced

2 to 3 tablespoons dressing of choice

Serves: 2   ◔ Cooking Time: 10 minutes

This simple green salad is an easy way to ensure there are vegetables at lunch or dinner. Vegetables are low in calories but high in vitamins, minerals, antioxidants, and fiber, all essential to maintain health and reduce the risk of chronic diseases.

1. Put the greens in a large bowl. Add the cucumber, cherry tomatoes, and red onion.

2. Drizzle on your dressing of choice a little at a time, tossing to mix, until the salad is dressed to your liking.

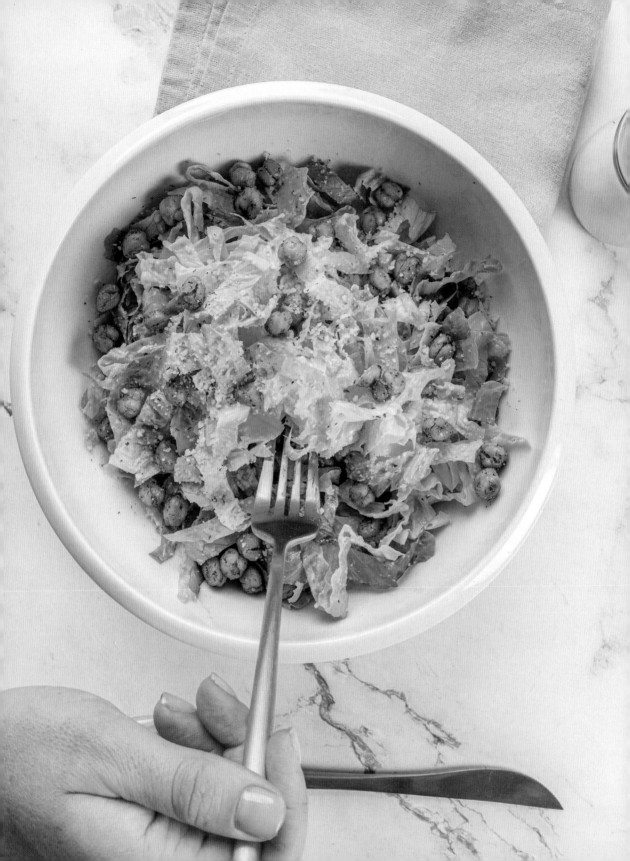

Chickpea "Caesar" Salad

Per 2 cups: Calories: 331 | Fat: 17g | Carbs: 34g | Fiber: 14g | Protein: 14g

2 heads romaine lettuce (about 4 cups, chopped)

2 batches Crispy Chickpeas (page 191)

1 batch Tahini Caesar Dressing (page 247)

½ cup Nutty "Cheese" Topper (page 237)

Black pepper, to taste

NOTES:

Add more veggies: Add cucumber, tomatoes, or bell peppers.

Serves: 4   🕐 Cooking Time: 10 minutes

Our take on a Caesar salad incorporates chickpeas, which are a great plant-based source of protein and fiber. Having chickpeas in place of an animal-based protein can help improve insulin sensitivity, so include them in your diet for blood-sugar benefits.

1. Place the lettuce and chickpeas in a large salad bowl and pour the dressing over the top. Top with the "cheese" and season with black pepper to taste. Mix well.

*Nutrition information is per serving

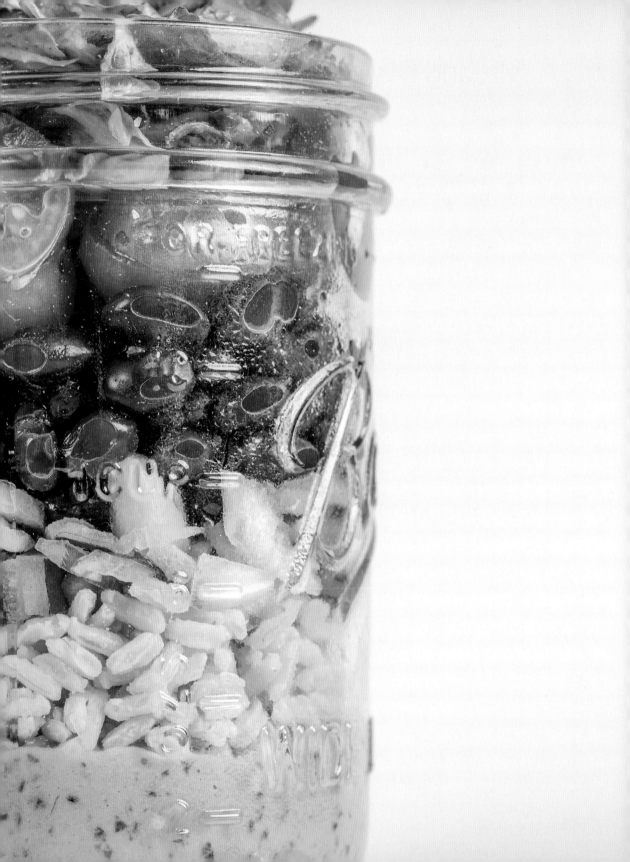

Mix-and-Match Mason Jar Salads

Serves: 1   Cooking Time: 5 minutes

DRESSING (PICK 1):
2–3 tablespoons

Creamy Orange-Ginger Dressing (page 245)

Creamy Balsamic Vinaigrette (page 244)

Tahini Caesar Dressing (page 247)

Green Goddess Drizzle (page 243)

Peanut Dipping Sauce (page 236)

Choose your own adventure with these mix-and-match mason jar salads. Select a variety of vegetables for a range of antioxidants, and pair them with a protein, whole grain, and the dressing of your choice. Mason jar salads are a great way to meal prep lunches for the week ahead. Modify the ingredients in this recipe based on what you have on hand or for more variety.

1. Layer your mason jar by adding the dressing first, followed by the whole grains, protein, and then the vegetables.

2. When ready to eat, shake the mason jar or pour the contents into a bowl and mix.

WHOLE GRAINS (PICK 1):
½–1 cup

Quinoa

Brown rice

Farro

Bulgur

Millet

Corn

VEGGIES (PICK 3): ½ cup each

Sliced cherry tomatoes

Shredded carrots

Cubed sweet potato

Diced cucumber

Shredded cabbage

Chopped mushrooms

Greens like romaine, spinach, kale, or arugula

NOTES:

Meal prep: keep mason jar salads in the fridge for up to four days.

Save time: Buy precooked grains and precut veggies.

Nutrition info will vary depending on selections.

PROTEIN (PICK 1): ½–1 cup

Black beans

Chickpeas

White beans

Kidney beans

Tofu

Lentils

Tempeh

Seitan

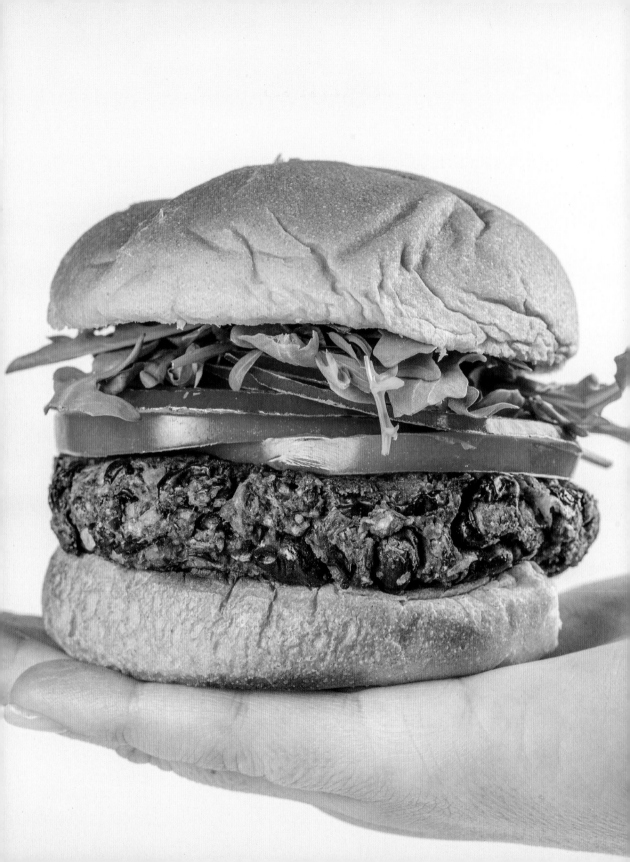

Mains

Curried Lentils with Kale and Cauliflower

Per 1½ cups: Calories: 228 | Fat: 5g | Carbs: 36g | Fiber: 9g | Protein: 13g

½ yellow onion, diced

2 garlic cloves, minced

1 tablespoon curry powder

½ teaspoon garam masala

½ teaspoon sea salt, divided

1 tablespoon tomato paste

2 cups vegetable stock, plus more
for sautéing

1 cup light canned coconut milk

¾ cup dried green lentils

1 head cauliflower, chopped into
small florets

2 cups chopped kale leaves,
stems removed

½ cup brown rice or quinoa, optional
(skip for a lower-carb option)

NOTES:

Store leftovers: Refrigerate in an
airtight container for up to five days.
Freeze for up to three months.

Save time: Buy precut cauliflower.

Serves: 4   ◔ Cooking Time: 40 minutes

Lentils are a fiber-rich, plant-based protein. This dish mixes them with
kale and cauliflower to provide even more fiber to help slow digestion
and regulate blood sugar.

1. In a pot over medium-high heat, sauté the onions with a few
splashes of vegetable stock. Cook until browned, about 3 to 5
minutes, stirring frequently and adding more stock as needed to
prevent the onions from sticking.

2. Add the garlic, curry powder, garam masala, ¼ teaspoon of the salt,
and the tomato paste. Stir for 1 minute.

3. Add the vegetable stock, coconut milk, and lentils. Bring to a
simmer and cook for 20 minutes uncovered. Add the cauliflower and
simmer for another 15 minutes, or until tender.

4. Stir in the kale leaves until wilted and season to taste with the
remaining ¼ teaspoon salt.

5. Serve with brown rice or quinoa, if desired.

*Nutrition information is per serving

Sweet Potato Black Bean Quinoa Bake

Per serving: Calories: 311 | Fat: 8g | Carbs: 52g | Fiber: 12g | Protein: 12g

1 ½ small sweet potatoes, chopped

1 cup cooked black beans

¾ cup quinoa

½ red bell pepper, chopped

2 green onions, chopped

2 ½ teaspoons chili powder

2 ½ teaspoons ground cumin

½ teaspoon garlic powder

⅛ teaspoon salt, or more to taste

1 cup vegetable stock

½ lime, juiced

½ avocado, diced

Serves: 3   🕐 Cooking Time: 55 minutes

Cooking the quinoa in the oven with vegetables and seasoning gives the dish more flavor and cuts time in the kitchen. The fiber from the quinoa, black beans, and sweet potato ensures this bake is blood sugar-friendly.

1. Preheat the oven to 375°F.

2. In a 8 x 8 inch baking dish, combine the sweet potatoes, black beans, quinoa, bell pepper, green onions, chili powder, cumin, garlic, and salt. Stir well to combine, then add the vegetable stock.

3. Cover the baking dish with foil and bake for 40 minutes, or until the stock has absorbed completely, the quinoa is fluffy, and the sweet potatoes are tender. Remove from the oven.

4. Let the quinoa bake sit for 5 minutes before serving. Top each plate with lime juice and avocado.

NOTES:

Store leftovers: Keeps well in the fridge for up to four days.

Save time: Buy precut sweet potatoes.

Add more flavor: Top with chopped cilantro.

Reduce food waste: Add leftover sweet potato to salads or bowls, or use in the Roasted Sweet Potato Salad with Arugula and Millet (page 145).

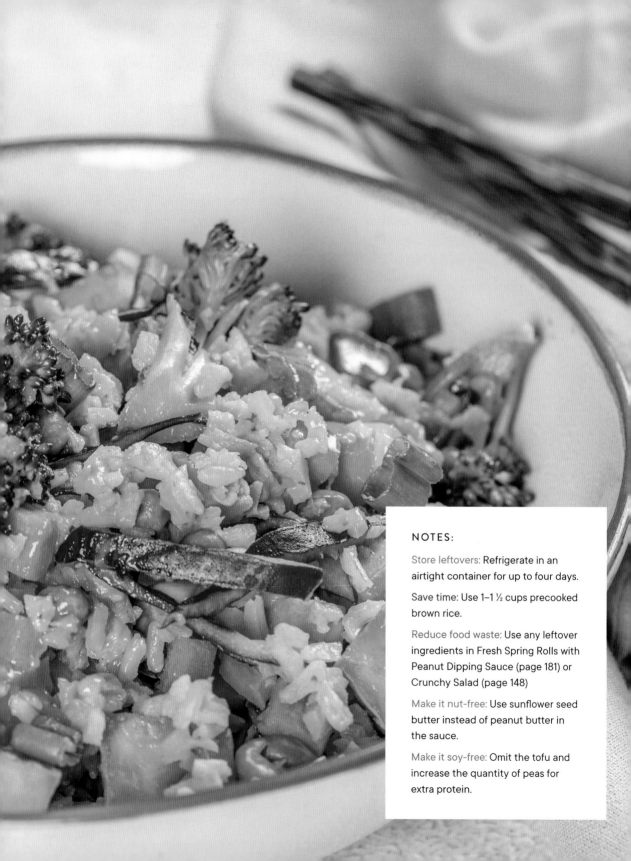

NOTES:

Store leftovers: Refrigerate in an airtight container for up to four days.

Save time: Use 1–1 ½ cups precooked brown rice.

Reduce food waste: Use any leftover ingredients in Fresh Spring Rolls with Peanut Dipping Sauce (page 181) or Crunchy Salad (page 148)

Make it nut-free: Use sunflower seed butter instead of peanut butter in the sauce.

Make it soy-free: Omit the tofu and increase the quantity of peas for extra protein.

Sticky Veggie Fried Rice

Per 2 cups: Calories: 382 | Fat: 14g | Carbs: 46g | Fiber: 9g | Protein: 24g

½ cup brown rice

1 (14-ounce) block tofu, extra firm, drained and pressed

½ teaspoon garlic powder

½ teaspoon onion powder

1 cup chopped green onions, divided into green and white parts

4 garlic cloves, minced

2 cups cauliflower rice, fresh or frozen

1 ½ cups shredded cabbage

1 cup finely diced carrots

½ cup peas, fresh or frozen

Sauce

¼ cup less-sodium soy sauce, tamari, or coconut aminos

2 tablespoons monk fruit sweetener

2 tablespoons peanut butter

1 garlic clove, minced

1 teaspoon fresh lime juice

½ teaspoon red pepper flakes

Serves: 3   🕐 Cooking Time: 45 minutes

Did you know the consumption of soy is associated with a decreased risk of type 2 diabetes? Tofu is an essential source of protein in a plant-based diet and excellent for people with diabetes. This veggie fried rice is a great way to add more tofu to the diet. Plus, adding cauliflower rice to this meal also helps add more fiber and volume with little impact on the total amount of carbohydrates.

1. Preheat the oven to 400°F and line a baking sheet with parchment paper.

2. Cook the rice according to the package instructions.

3. Once the oven is preheated, dice the tofu into ¼-inch cubes and toss them with the garlic and onion powder.

4. Arrange the tofu on the baking sheet and bake for 25 minutes, or until the tofu is crisp and firm to the touch.

5. While the tofu cooks, prepare the sauce by mixing all the ingredients in a bowl and whisking until well combined.

6. Heat a large nonstick skillet or wok (or a pan lightly sprayed with olive oil cooking spray) over medium heat. Add the white parts of the green onions and the garlic and cook for 1–2 minutes, stirring occasionally.

7. Add the cauliflower rice, cabbage, carrots, and peas. Cook for 3–4 minutes, stirring occasionally.

8. Add the brown rice, tofu, and sauce to the pan and stir to combine.

9. Top with the green parts of the green onions when ready to serve.

Mushroom Black Bean Burgers

Per patty: Calories: 189 | Fat: 5g | Carbs: 26g | Fiber: 10g | Protein: 11g

1 ½ cups mushrooms, chopped

½ yellow or white onion, finely chopped

2 garlic cloves, minced

2 cups cooked black beans

Juice of 1 lime

½ cup fresh cilantro, chopped

¼ cup ground flaxseed

½ teaspoon red pepper flakes

½ teaspoon salt

¼ teaspoon black pepper

¼ teaspoon ground cumin

1 tablespoon ketchup, Eggless Mayo (page 240), or store-bought vegan mayonnaise

NOTES:

Reduce food waste: Toss leftover black beans, onion, and mushrooms into your next salad or wrap. Or use these ingredients in the Black Bean Quesadillas with Cashew Nacho "Cheese" Sauce (page 184).

No black beans? Use kidney or pinto beans instead.

Store leftovers: Store uncooked or cooked black bean patties in the freezer for up to three months.

Makes 4   🕐 Cooking Time: 40 minutes

Replacing red meat with plant-based proteins, as in this black bean burger recipe, can reduce insulin resistance and improve blood sugar levels. Filled with black beans and ground flaxseed, these burgers are rich in fiber and low in saturated fat. The mushrooms also help to add texture, depth, and additional nutrients to the patties.

1. In a nonstick cooking pan (or a pan lightly sprayed with olive oil cooking spray), sauté the mushrooms, onion, and garlic over medium heat for 3–5 minutes, or until the onions are translucent.

2. Place the beans in a large bowl and mash with a potato masher, leaving some chunks throughout the mixture for texture.

3. Add the mushroom mixture and all the remaining ingredients to the beans. Mix until everything is well combined.

4. Refrigerate the mixture for 15 minutes.

5. Shape the mixture into four separate balls, then press each one down using the palm of your hand or the bottom of a cup until it forms the shape of a burger patty.

6. Heat a nonstick cooking pan (or a pan lightly sprayed with olive oil cooking spray) over medium heat.

7. Once the pan is hot, add the burgers and cook for about 7 minutes on each side, or until a nice golden crust forms.

8. Let cool for 10 minutes before serving.

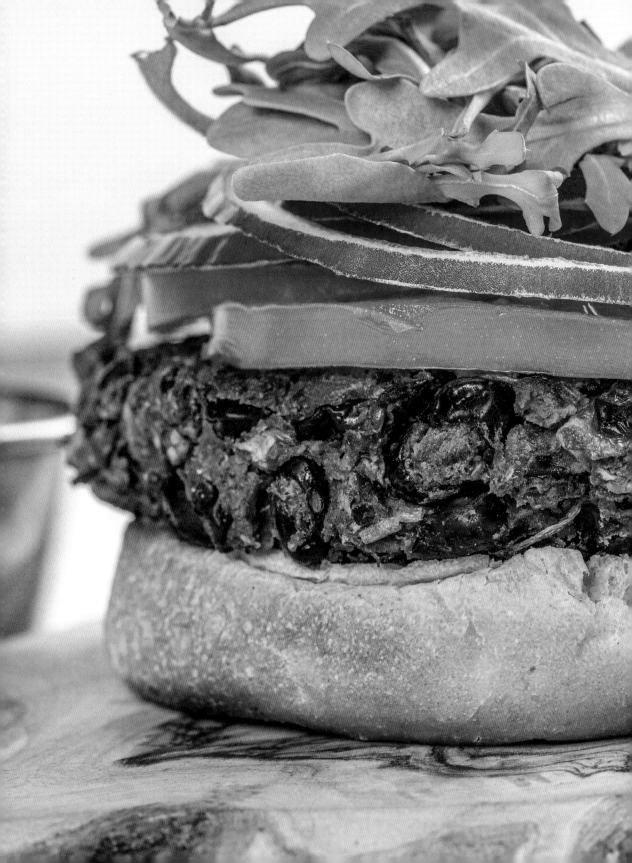

Spaghetti Squash with Lentil "No Meat" Sauce

Per ⅓ squash and 1 cup lentil sauce: Calories: 254 | Fat: 10g | Carbs: 37g | Fiber: 9g | Protein: 9g

1 large spaghetti squash

Salt and black pepper, to taste

1 batch Lentil "No Meat" Sauce (page 220)

Nutty "Cheese" Topper (page 237), optional

NOTES:

No spaghetti squash? Use zucchini noodles or bean pasta instead.

Reduce food waste: Save the spaghetti squash seeds, season, and roast at 425°F until toasted and crunchy.

Serves: 3   ◷ Cooking Time: 1 hour

This lentil tomato sauce is reminiscent of a Bolognese, but without the saturated fat and with more fiber. Add in the spaghetti squash, and this dish becomes a great meat-sauce replacement that is highly beneficial for your long-term blood sugar.

1. Preheat the oven to 400°F and line a baking sheet with parchment paper.

2. Cut the spaghetti squash in half lengthwise and scoop out the seeds. Coat the cut side of the squash (the flesh side) with olive oil cooking spray and sprinkle with salt and pepper.

3. Place the squash on the baking sheet, flesh side down so the skin is facing up. Bake for 30–40 minutes, or until the squash is soft and stringy and can be pulled with a fork.

4. Once the squash is done, remove it from the oven and flip the squash so that it's cut side up. When cool to the touch, use a fork to scrape and fluff the strands from the sides of the squash.

5. Top with the lentil bolognese sauce and serve with the nutty "cheese" topper, if desired.

*Nutrition information is per serving

Tofu Crumble Tacos

Per 2 tacos: Calories: 305 | Fat: 13g | Carbs: 29g | Fiber: 8g | Protein: 25g

1 (14-ounce) block tofu, extra firm, drained and pressed

2 tablespoons less-sodium soy sauce or tamari

1 tablespoon chili powder

¾ teaspoon ground cumin

½ teaspoon salt

½ teaspoon dried oregano

¼ teaspoon garlic powder

¼ teaspoon onion powder

½ cup tomato sauce

4 (6-inch) corn or whole-wheat flour tortillas and/or romaine lettuce leaves

OPTIONAL TOPPINGS:

Guacamole

Cashew Sour Cream (page 241)

Shredded lettuce

Chopped tomatoes

NOTES:

Add more vegetables: Add zucchini, onions, or broccoli.

Make it gluten-free: Use corn or gluten-free tortillas.

Make it soy-free: Use lentils in place of tofu and use coconut aminos in place of soy sauce.

Serves: 2   🕐 Cooking Time: 20 minutes

These tofu crumble tacos make an excellent replacement for ground beef tacos, which can contain well over 12 grams of saturated fat per serving. By replacing meat for tofu, we slashed the saturated fat content to just 2 grams. Top the tacos with different vegetables for an extra boost of fiber and even more blood sugar benefits.

1. Crumble the tofu into a large nonstick skillet (or a skillet lightly sprayed with olive oil cooking spray) over medium heat.

2. Add all the remaining ingredients except for the tomato sauce and tortillas, and stir to combine. Continue cooking until most of the liquid has evaporated from the tofu, 10–15 minutes. Add the tomato sauce and cook for an additional 5 minutes.

3. Fill tortillas or lettuce wraps with the tofu "meat" and serve with any other desired toppings.

Penne Pesto with Spinach and Cherry Tomatoes

Per serving: Calories: 494 | Fat: 18g | Carbs: 71g | Fiber: 16g | Protein: 18g

8 ounces 100% whole-wheat penne

2 cups cherry tomatoes

Pinch of salt

2 tablespoons balsamic vinegar

2 cups spinach

1 cup Basil Spinach Pesto (page 223)

1 (15-ounce) can white beans, drained and rinsed

Nutritional yeast and red pepper flakes, optional

NOTES:

No white beans? Skip the beans and use bean pasta instead of whole-wheat.

Add more vegetables: Add in any leftover cooked vegetables, such as peppers, onions, or zucchini.

Make it gluten-free: Use quinoa, rice, or bean pasta instead of the whole-wheat penne.

Serves: 4   ● Cooking Time: 15 minutes

Don't let the high-carbohydrate content of pasta stop you from enjoying this delicious food. Pasta can absolutely be part of a whole-food, plant-based diet for diabetes. While this meal may contain a high amount of carbs, the whole-wheat pasta, beans, and veggies help to boost the protein and fiber content, making it more favorable for blood sugar.

1. Cook the pasta according to the package instructions.

2. While the pasta is cooking, heat a small saucepan over medium heat. Add a splash of water, the tomatoes, and the salt and cook until the tomatoes burst, 3–5 minutes. Add the balsamic vinegar and stir.

3. Place the spinach in a colander. When the pasta is ready, set aside ½ cup of the pasta water, then drain the pasta over the spinach to slightly wilt it. Mix the reserved pasta water with the pesto.

4. In a bowl, combine the pasta, tomatoes, pesto, and white beans and mix until they are well combined.

5. Serve topped with nutritional yeast and red pepper flakes, if desired.

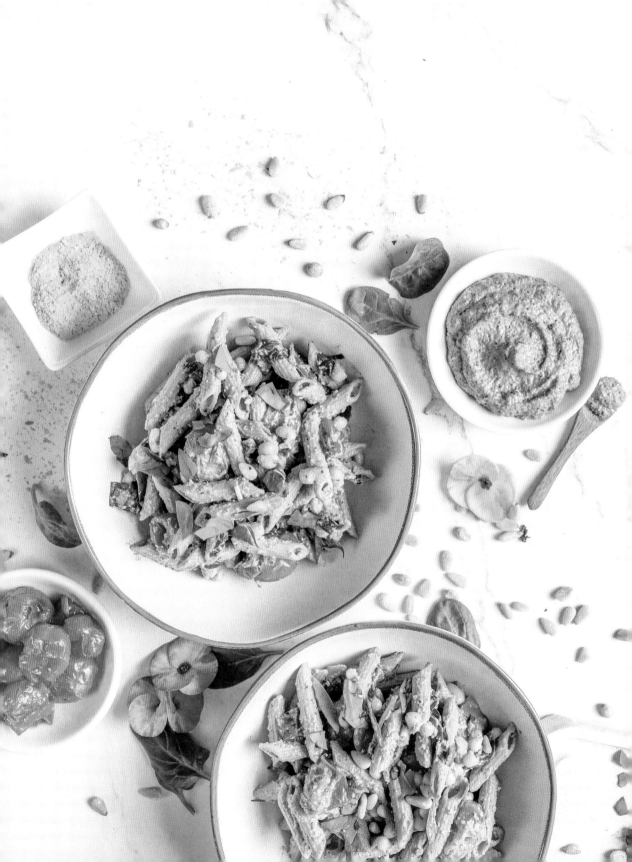

One-Pan Chickpeas with Rainbow Veggies

Per serving: Calories: 301 | Fat: 4g | Carbs: 55g | Fiber: 15g | Protein: 16g

2 cups cherry tomatoes

1 yellow bell pepper, sliced

2 cups chopped broccoli (chopped into small florets)

1 red onion, chopped

1 (15-ounce) can chickpeas, drained and rinsed

Salt and black pepper, to taste

Green Goddess Drizzle (page 243), Creamy Balsamic Vinaigrette (page 244), or Creamy Orange-Ginger Dressing (page 245), optional

Whole grains of choice (like brown rice, quinoa, or farro), optional

NOTES:

No chickpeas? Use marinated tofu, black beans, or lentils.

Store leftovers: Keeps well in the fridge for two to three days.

Save time: Buy precut veggies to save time chopping.

Serves: 2   🕐 Cooking Time: 40 minutes

One-pan meals are quick to put together, making them a convenient weeknight dinner. By eating an array of different-colored vegetables in the recipe, you're also consuming many phytonutrients—the pigments that give fruits and vegetables their color. Phytonutrients are linked to higher levels of specific nutrients and many health benefits.

1. Preheat the oven to 375°F and line a baking sheet with parchment paper.

2. Place the cherry tomatoes, bell pepper, broccoli, red onion, and chickpeas on the baking sheet. Spray with olive oil cooking spray and sprinkle with salt and pepper.

3. Place in the oven and bake for 30 minutes.

4. Serve with whole grains and your dressing of choice, if desired.

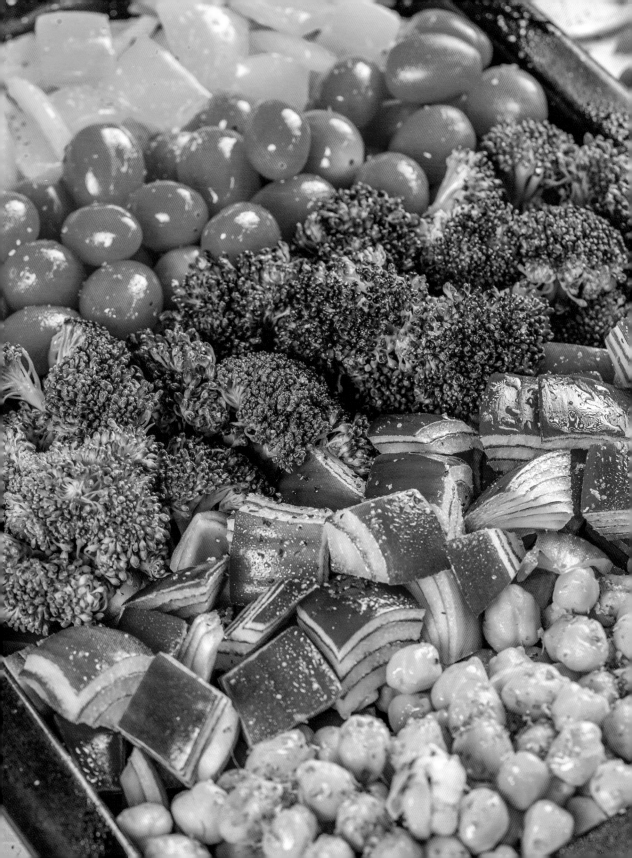

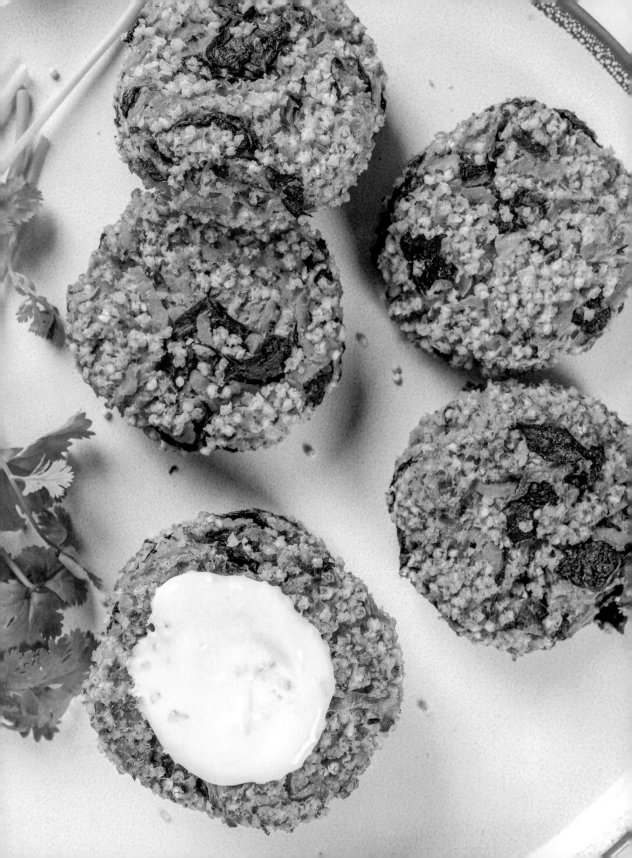

Veggie-Packed Millet Cakes with Dipping Sauce

Per 2 cakes + 2 tablespoons dip: Calories: 184 | Fat: 5g | Carbs: 30g | Fiber: 6g | Protein: 7g

1 cup millet, rinsed

½ small onion, diced

2 garlic cloves, minced

8 cups spinach, roughly chopped

3 large carrots, peeled and grated

2 teaspoons curry powder

¾ teaspoon salt

½ teaspoon black pepper

¼ cup unsweetened, plain non-dairy yogurt

¼ cup ground flaxseed

2 tablespoons minced fresh cilantro

Dip

1 cup unsweetened, plain non-dairy yogurt

Juice of ½ lemon

¼ teaspoon salt

¼ teaspoon black pepper

¼ teaspoon red pepper flakes

NOTES:

Plan ahead: Make a big batch of millet cakes and freeze before baking for future meals.

Save time: Cook the millet in an Instant Pot® or other electric multi-cooker.

Makes 14   🕐 Cooking Time: 1 hour 45 minutes

Millet is an ancient grain that is naturally gluten-free and high in protein and fiber. Regular consumption of millet has been shown to reduce blood sugar levels and improve insulin resistance. These veggie-packed millet cakes are a fun and unique way to consume more millet!

1. Preheat the oven to 400°F and line a baking sheet with parchment paper.

2. While the oven is preheating, combine the millet with 2 cups water in a saucepan over medium heat and bring to a boil.

3. Reduce the heat to a simmer, cover, and cook for 15 minutes, until the liquid is absorbed. Turn off the heat and let the millet sit in the pot for 10 more minutes.

4. Place the cooked millet in a large mixing bowl and set aside to cool.

5. In a nonstick pan (or a pan lightly sprayed with olive oil cooking spray), cook the onion and garlic over medium heat, stirring frequently until the onions are soft and translucent, 3–5 minutes.

6. Add the spinach, carrots, curry powder, salt, and pepper. Cook and stir for about 2 minutes.

7. Add the vegetables to the millet, then add the yogurt, flaxseed, and cilantro and stir until evenly combined.

8. Use a ⅓-cup measure to make ½-inch-thick round patties and place them on the baking sheet. Refrigerate for 20 minutes.

9. Bake the cakes for 25–30 minutes, or until the cakes are crispy and cooked through.

10. While the cakes are cooking, combine all the ingredients for the dip in a small bowl.

11. Serve the cakes warm out of the oven with the dip.

*Nutrition information is per serving

Pinto Bean Fajitas

Per 2 fajitas: Calories: 335 | Fat: 3g | Carbs: 65g | Fiber: 17g | Protein: 16g

½ small yellow onion, sliced

1 red bell pepper, sliced

1 yellow bell pepper, sliced

2 garlic cloves, minced

1 teaspoon chili powder

1 teaspoon ground cumin

½ teaspoon salt

¼–½ teaspoon chipotle or cayenne powder, optional

1 (15-ounce) can pinto beans, drained and rinsed

4 (6-inch) corn or whole-wheat flour tortillas and/or romaine lettuce leaves

OPTIONAL TOPPINGS:

Guacamole

Cashew Sour Cream (page 241)

Shredded lettuce

Chopped tomatoes

NOTES:

Make it gluten-free: **Use corn tortillas or lettuce leaves.**

Serves: 2   🕐 Cooking Time: 20 minutes

Loaded with pinto beans and veggies, these easy Pinto Bean Fajitas are the perfect way to get a delicious and healthy meal on the table in minutes! Pinto beans also contain protein, fiber, and important vitamins, and minerals such as thiamine (a B-vitamin), iron, magnesium, and potassium.

1. In a large nonstick skillet (or a skillet lightly sprayed with olive oil cooking spray), combine the onions and bell peppers over medium-high heat and cook for 6–7 minutes, stirring occasionally.

2. Add the garlic, chili powder, cumin, salt, and chipotle or cayenne, if using, and cook for 1 minute more.

3. Add the beans and cook until heated through, about 3 more minutes.

4. Fill the tortillas or lettuce wraps with the bean mixture and serve with any other desired toppings.

Breaded Tofu "Fish" Fingers

Per ⅓ serving of breaded tofu and 2 tablespoons vegan aioli:
Calories: 475 | Fat: 35g | Carbs: 327g | Fiber: 4g | Protein: 17g

½ cup cornstarch

2 tablespoons nutritional yeast

1 tablespoon garlic powder

1 tablespoon onion powder

3 teaspoons Old Bay
seasoning, divided

1 ½ teaspoons salt, divided

¾ teaspoon black pepper, divided

½ cup unsweetened non-dairy milk

1 tablespoon apple cider vinegar

½ cup whole-wheat breadcrumbs

1 (14-ounce) block tofu, extra firm,
drained and pressed

SPICY VEGAN AIOLI SAUCE

½ cup Eggless Mayo (page 240) or
store-bought vegan mayonnaise

1 tablespoon sriracha

½ teaspoon garlic powder

NOTES:

Serve it up: Serve with a side salad,
or in lettuce wraps with a side of
cooked veggies.

Make it gluten-free: Use corn tortillas
or lettuce leaves. Use cornmeal
instead of the breadcrumbs.

Make it soy-free: Use seitan instead
of the tofu.

Serves: 3   ⏱ Cooking Time: 55 minutes

Even tofu-skeptics will love this recipe! Our fish-free version of fish fingers is a great recipe to cook and enjoy with kids. Cornstarch helps make tofu extra crispy, whole-wheat bread crumbs adds more fiber to this dish, and baking them in the oven saves on calories and fat. They are easy to whip up and kid-approved!

1. Preheat the oven to 425°F.

2. In one bowl, combine the cornstarch, nutritional yeast, garlic powder, onion powder, 2 teaspoons of the Old Bay seasoning, 1 teaspoon of the salt, and ½ teaspoon of the pepper. Whisk everything together. Add the non-dairy milk and apple cider vinegar and whisk together to form a wet batter. Let sit for 5 minutes.

3. In a second bowl, combine the whole-wheat breadcrumbs with the remaining 1 teaspoon of Old Bay seasoning, ½ teaspoon salt, and ¼ teaspoon pepper. Mix together.

4. Slice the tofu into ¾-inch-thick slabs.

5. Place a tofu slice in the first bowl of wet batter and cover it completely, then dip it in the breadcrumb mixture and cover completely.

6. Place the breaded tofu slice on a baking sheet. Repeat with all the remaining tofu.

7. Place the breaded tofu in the oven and bake for 25 minutes, or until golden brown. Remove from the oven and let cool.

8. Meanwhile, combine all the ingredients for the aioli in a small bowl.

9. Serve the breaded tofu "fish" fingers with the aioli on top. Enjoy!

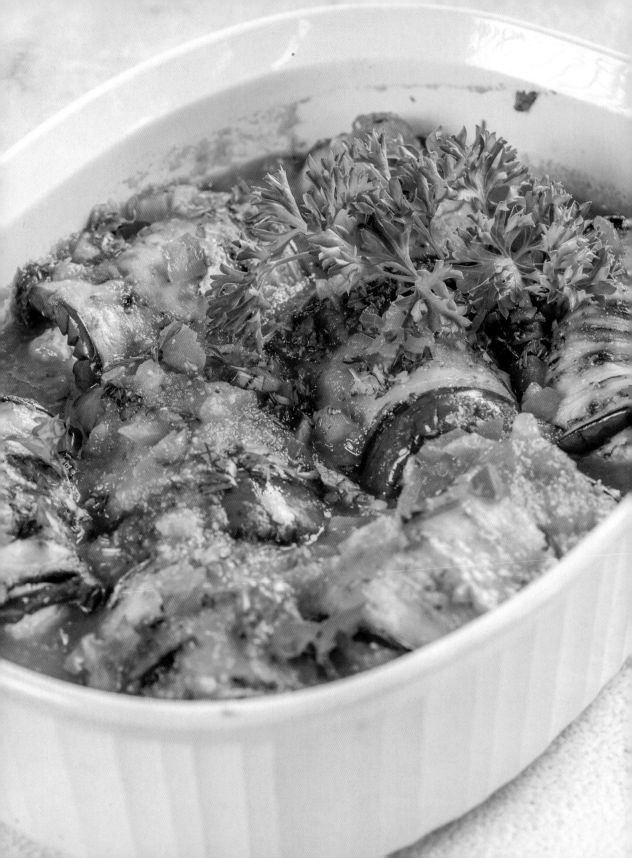

Eggplant "Ricotta" Roll-Ups

Per 3 roll-ups: Calories: 210 | Fat: 7g | Carbs: 29g | Fiber: 13g | Protein: 18g

1 large eggplant

A few pinches of salt

½ batch (1 ½ cups) Herbed "Ricotta" Filling (page 221)

1 cup Fresh Basil Tomato Sauce (page 224) or store-bought tomato sauce

Whole-wheat or bean pasta, optional

NOTES:

No eggplant? Use zucchini instead.

Make it soy-free: Use a cashew-based "ricotta" filling.

Serves: 2   ◷ Cooking Time: 30 minutes

Eggplants are rich in polyphenols, compounds found in plants that help mitigate stress and inflammation in the body. Moreover, polyphenols may influence carbohydrate metabolism, encouraging greater removal of glucose (blood sugar) from the bloodstream and contributing to improved insulin sensitivity.

1. Preheat the oven to 375°F.

2. While the oven preheats, slice the eggplant into ½-inch-thick slices, lay the slices on a layer of paper towels, and sprinkle generously with salt to remove excess moisture. Pat dry.

3. In a nonstick skillet (or a skillet lightly sprayed with olive oil cooking spray), cook the eggplant slices for 1–2 minutes on each side, or until they are soft enough for rolling up.

4. Place each eggplant slice on a plate or baking sheet, place a heaping spoonful of the tofu ricotta mixture on one side, and gently roll it up.

5. Spread ½ cup of the tomato sauce in an 8 x 8 inch baking dish, add the rolled-up eggplant bundles, then top with the remaining ½ cup tomato sauce.

6. Bake in the oven for about 20 minutes.

7. Serve with whole-wheat or bean pasta, if desired.

*Nutrition information is per serving

Stuffed Peppers with Lentils

Per 1 pepper with approximately 1 cup filling: Calories: 255 | Fat: 2g | Carbs: 47g | Fiber: 9g | Protein: 14g

1 small yellow onion, chopped

3 garlic cloves, minced, divided

1 teaspoon ground cumin

1 teaspoon paprika

1 teaspoon dried oregano

½ teaspoon salt, plus more for the peppers

¼ teaspoon red pepper flakes

½ cup dried brown lentils

½ cup quinoa

1 medium tomato, chopped

1 ½ cups vegetable stock, plus more for sautéing

4 large red bell peppers, cored and sliced in half

Black pepper, to taste

2 tablespoons chopped fresh cilantro or parsley

Sliced avocado or a dollop of Cashew Sour Cream (page 241), optional

Serves: 4   🕐 Cooking Time: 1 hour and 15 minutes

Lentils are a great plant-based source of iron, which is essential for carrying oxygen from the lungs to the tissues in the body. Pairing iron with a source of vitamin C—such as the red peppers in this recipe—aids its absorption.

1. Preheat the oven to 375°F and line a baking sheet with parchment paper.

2. While the oven preheats, heat a few splashes of vegetable stock in a medium pot over medium heat. Add the onion, 2 garlic cloves, the cumin, paprika, oregano, salt, and red pepper flakes and cook, stirring frequently, until the onions become translucent, 3–5 minutes. Add more vegetable stock as needed to prevent the onions from browning.

3. Add the lentils, quinoa, tomato, and vegetable stock. Bring the mixture to a boil, then reduce the heat to low. Cover and simmer for 30 minutes, or until the lentils are tender and the quinoa is cooked. Stir once halfway through, then again toward the end of the cooking time. If the mixture looks too dry, splash in additional stock or water.

4. While the lentil-quinoa mixture cooks, lightly spray the peppers with olive oil cooking spray and season with salt, pepper, and the remaining minced garlic. Place the peppers cut side up on the baking sheet.

5. Fill the peppers with the lentil mix and cover the tray with foil.

6. Bake for 30 minutes, then remove the foil and increase the oven temperature to 400°F. Cook for another 15 minutes, until the peppers are slightly browned and soft. Remove from the oven.

7. Top with the chopped fresh cilantro or parsley and serve with sliced avocado or Cashew Sour Cream, if desired.

*Nutrition information is per serving

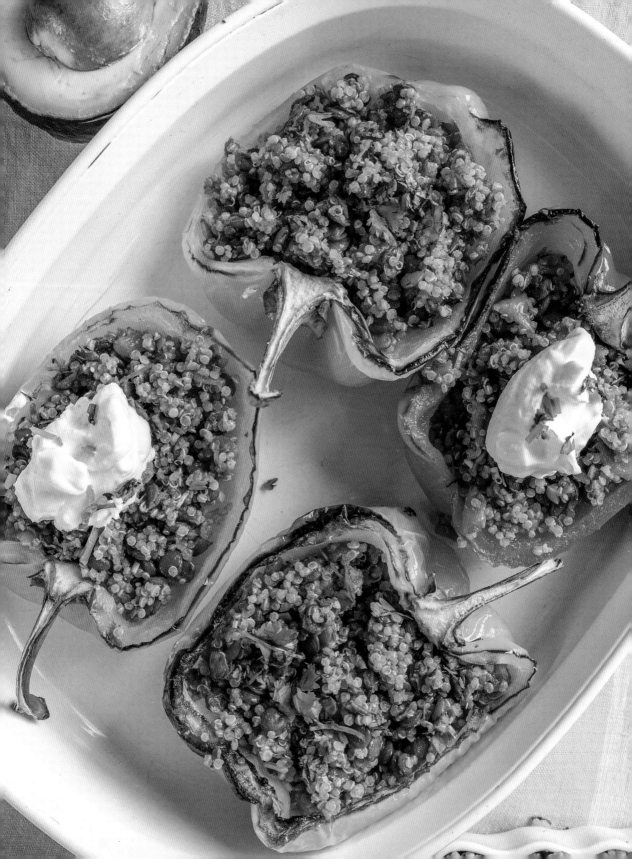

Teriyaki Tempeh and Broccoli Stir-Fry

Per serving: Calories: 291 | Fat: 13g | Carbs: 22g | Fiber: 4g | Protein: 29g

1 (8-ounce) package tempeh, cut into ¼-inch strips

¼ cup vegetable stock, plus more as needed

3 cups broccoli florets

4 garlic cloves, minced

Teriyaki Sauce

3 tablespoons less-sodium soy sauce or tamari

2 tablespoons vegetable stock

½ tablespoon monk fruit sweetener

2 garlic cloves, minced

½ teaspoon grated fresh ginger

Brown rice or cauliflower rice, optional

Serves: 2   🕐 Cooking Time: 20 minutes

Typical teriyaki dishes can be sneaky sources of added sugar and salt. This version keeps the sugar low by using monk fruit to sweeten the sauce, and opts for a less-sodium tamari to help control the salt.

1. In a small bowl, combine the teriyaki sauce ingredients and whisk until well combined. Set aside.

2. In a large skillet, combine the tempeh and vegetable stock over medium-low heat. Cook the tempeh for about 5 minutes on each side, or until golden brown. Add more vegetable stock as needed to prevent the tempeh from burning.

3. Add the teriyaki sauce, broccoli, and garlic to the pan and sauté for another 10 minutes, or until the broccoli is tender, mixing occasionally.

4. Serve with brown rice or cauliflower rice, if desired.

NOTES:

Make it soy-free: Use seitan or lentils in place of the tempeh. Use coconut aminos in place of the soy sauce.

Baked Falafel

Per 4 falafel balls: Calories: 281 | Fat: 4g | Carbs: 48g | Fiber: 10g | Protein: 15g

2 cups dried chickpeas

2 teaspoons baking soda

3 shallots, roughly chopped

1 cup fresh parsley, stems removed

8 garlic cloves

1 ½ tsp ground cumin

1 ½ teaspoon ground coriander

1 ½ teaspoon paprika

1 teaspoon salt

1 teaspoon black pepper

½ teaspoon cayenne pepper

NOTES:

Serve it up: Enjoy with brown rice and/or a salad and our Lebanese-Style Cucumber Yogurt Sauce (page 235).

Serves: 6   ◷ Cooking Time: 50 minutes

Falafel is a popular Middle Eastern food made with chickpeas, herbs, and spices, and is traditionally deep fried in oil. In our version, we bake the falafel, which helps to significantly decrease the calorie and fat content. These falafel make an excellent source of plant-protein and come packed with antioxidants from the herbs and spices.

1. In a large bowl, combine the chickpeas and baking soda, and fill with water until the chickpeas are covered by at least 2 inches. Soak overnight for 18 hours or longer. When ready, drain the chickpeas and pat them dry.

2. Preheat the oven to 350°F and line a 9 x 12-inch glass baking dish with parchment paper or spray with olive oil cooking spray.

3. In a food processor, puree the chickpeas, then add the remaining ingredients and puree into a homogenous paste.

4. Using your hands, shape the paste into ½-inch thick balls. Place the balls in a single layer in the prepared baking dish and spray with olive oil cooking spray.

5. Bake the falafel for 30 minutes, or until golden brown, turning over midway through. Serve warm.

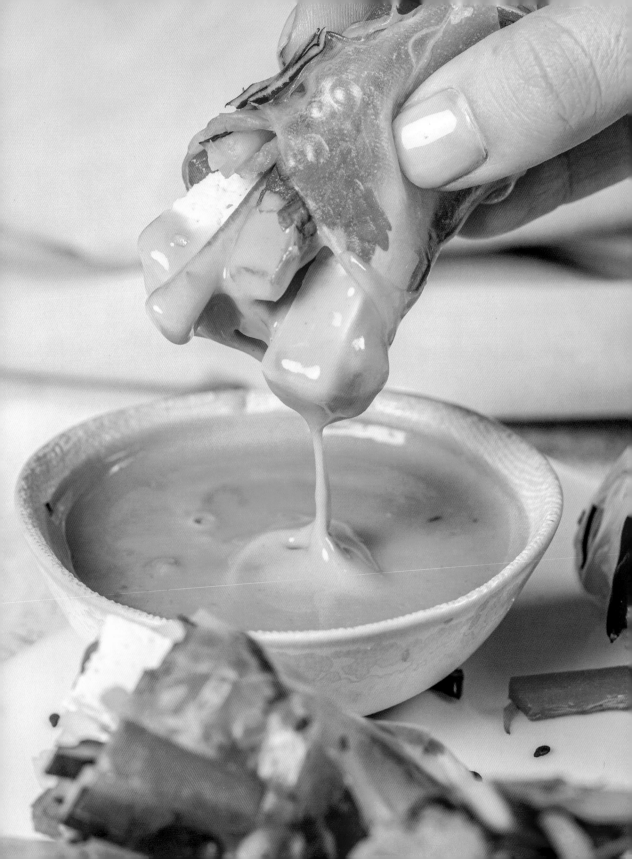

Fresh Spring Rolls with Peanut Dipping Sauce

Per 3 spring rolls and 3 tablespoons sauce: Calories: 315 | Fat: 14g | Carbs: 38g | Fiber: 4g | Protein: 15g

1 (14-ounce) block tofu, extra firm, drained and pressed

12 spring roll rice paper wrappers

2 medium carrots, cut into matchsticks

1 cup shredded cabbage

1 bell pepper, cut into matchsticks

1 cucumber, cut into matchsticks

¼ cup chopped cilantro

1 batch Peanut Dipping Sauce (page 236)

NOTES:

Add more carbs: Add brown rice vermicelli noodles.

Shop smart: Spring roll rice paper wrappers are generally found in the Asian foods section at the grocery store.

Serves: 4   🕐 Cooking Time: 1 hour

Spring rolls can be a fun and convenient way to eat the rainbow. These spring rolls contain five different vegetables and herbs, providing you with a variety of antioxidants. Consuming an antioxidant-rich diet can help improve insulin sensitivity.

1. Preheat the oven to 400°F. Line a baking sheet with parchment paper.

2. Slice the tofu into ½-inch strips and arrange on the baking sheet. Bake for 25 minutes, or until the tofu is crisp and firm to the touch.

3. Fill a large bowl or plate with water. Dip a sheet of rice paper into the water for 10–15 seconds until the paper becomes soft and malleable. Remove from the water and place on a flat surface.

4. On one end of the rice paper, layer a small amount of the tofu, vegetables, and cilantro.

5. Fold in the sides of the rice paper, then begin rolling it away from you, as you would a burrito. Continue rolling all the way up.

6. Repeat steps 3–5 with the remaining rice papers. Serve with the peanut sauce.

Pasta Primavera

Per 1½ cups: Calories: 265 | Fat: 4g | Carbs: 48g | Fiber: 12g | Protein: 18g

8 ounces chickpea or lentil pasta

½ medium red onion, sliced

6 garlic cloves, minced

½ teaspoon salt, plus more to taste

½ tablespoon dried oregano or Italian seasoning

1 cup sliced broccoli florets

½ medium yellow bell pepper, sliced into matchsticks

1 medium yellow squash, cut into half moons

1 medium zucchini, cut into half moons

2 cups Fresh Basil Tomato Sauce (page 224) or store-bought pasta sauce

¼ cup fresh parsley

Black pepper, to taste

Nutty "Cheese" Topper (page 237), optional

Serves: 4   🕐 Cooking Time: 25 minutes

Bean-based pastas increase the fiber and protein content of a meal, making them ideal for blood sugar management. Pairing bean pasta with lots of veggies, as in this pasta primavera, increases the fiber and water content of the meal, contributing to even more satiety.

1. Prepare the pasta according to the package instructions.

2. Meanwhile, in a nonstick pan (or a pan lightly sprayed with olive oil cooking spray), cook the red onion, garlic, salt, and oregano over medium heat for 2–3 minutes, stirring frequently.

3. Add the broccoli and bell peppers to the pan and cook for another 2–3 minutes, then add the squash and zucchini and cook until all the vegetables have softened, about 5 minutes.

4. In a large bowl, combine the pasta, sautéed vegetables, and tomato sauce. Mix well until the pasta is coated with the sauce.

5. Adjust the salt and pepper based on your preferences. Serve sprinkled with the fresh parsley and nutty cheese topper, if desired.

*Nutrition information is per serving

Veggie Pad Thai Noodles

Per 1½ cups: Calories: 312 | Fat: 8g | Carbs: 50g | Fiber: 9g | Protein: 14g

6 ounces brown rice noodles

¼ cup vegetable stock

3 garlic cloves, minced

2 cups chopped broccoli florets

1 medium carrot, peeled and shaved into noodle-like strands (use a vegetable peeler)

1 red bell pepper, seeded and sliced

½ red onion, sliced

1½ cups shelled edamame, frozen

1 cup shredded purple cabbage

¼ cup crushed peanuts

3 green onions, chopped

Sauce

3 tablespoons less-sodium soy sauce or tamari

2 tablespoons monk fruit sweetener

2 tablespoons rice vinegar

2 tablespoons fresh lime juice

1 teaspoon sriracha

Serves: 4   ◷ Cooking Time: 35 minutes

This homemade veggie pad Thai uses brown rice noodles to boost the dish's fiber content. The array of vegetables adds volume and nutrients, helping to fill you up and keep you satiated.

1. Cook the rice noodles according to the package instructions, then rinse under cold water to prevent sticking and set aside.

2. In a large frying pan, combine the vegetable stock, minced garlic, and the red onion. Sauté over medium heat until fragrant, about 2 minutes.

3. Add the broccoli, carrots, bell peppers, edamame, and cabbage to the pan and cook for 6 minutes, stirring frequently.

4. Meanwhile, in a small bowl, whisk together all the ingredients for the sauce and set aside.

5. After all the vegetables are cooked and soft, add the rice noodles to the pan and mix everything together.

6. Pour the sauce into the pan and stir to coat all of the noodles and vegetables.

7. Top with green onion and crushed peanuts.

NOTES:

Make it soy-free: Swap the edamame for lima beans (usually found in the freezer section of the grocery store) and use coconut aminos in place of soy sauce.

Black Bean Quesadillas with Cashew Nacho "Cheese" Sauce

Per quesadilla: Calories: 409 | Fat: 15g | Carbs: 55g | Fiber: 17g | Protein: 18g

2 (10-inch) whole-wheat tortillas

½ small onion, diced

½ red bell pepper, diced

6 small mushrooms, sliced

2 cups chopped spinach

1 cup cooked black beans

2 garlic cloves, minced

½ teaspoon paprika

½ teaspoon chili powder

½ teaspoon salt

¼ teaspoon black pepper

¼ teaspoon ground cumin

⅓ cup Cashew Nacho "Cheese" Sauce (page 232)

NOTES:

Reduce food waste: Use leftover onion, bell pepper, mushrooms, and black beans in a salad or wrap.

No black beans? Use kidney, pinto, or red beans instead.

Make it gluten-free: Use gluten-free or corn tortillas.

Serves: 2   🕐 Cooking Time: 25 minutes

Yes, quesadillas can be part of a blood sugar-friendly eating pattern! Adding black beans, mushrooms, peppers, and spinach to the quesadilla increases its fiber content. And using cashew "cheese" instead of regular cheese lowers the saturated fat content, making this quesadilla an all-around good choice for blood sugar management.

1. In a nonstick pan (or a pan lightly sprayed with olive oil cooking spray), cook the onion over medium heat for 2–3 minutes, then add the peppers and mushrooms and cook for another 2–3 minutes, until soft, stirring often.

2. Add the spinach, black beans, garlic, paprika, chili powder, salt, pepper, and cumin to the pan and mix to combine. Cook just until all the ingredients are heated through.

3. Place one tortilla in a nonstick pan over medium heat. Spread half of the Cashew Nacho "Cheese" Sauce over one side of the tortilla, then add half the filling. Fold the other side of the tortilla over to enclose the filling, and fry on both sides until golden. Repeat with the second tortilla.

*Nutrition information is per serving

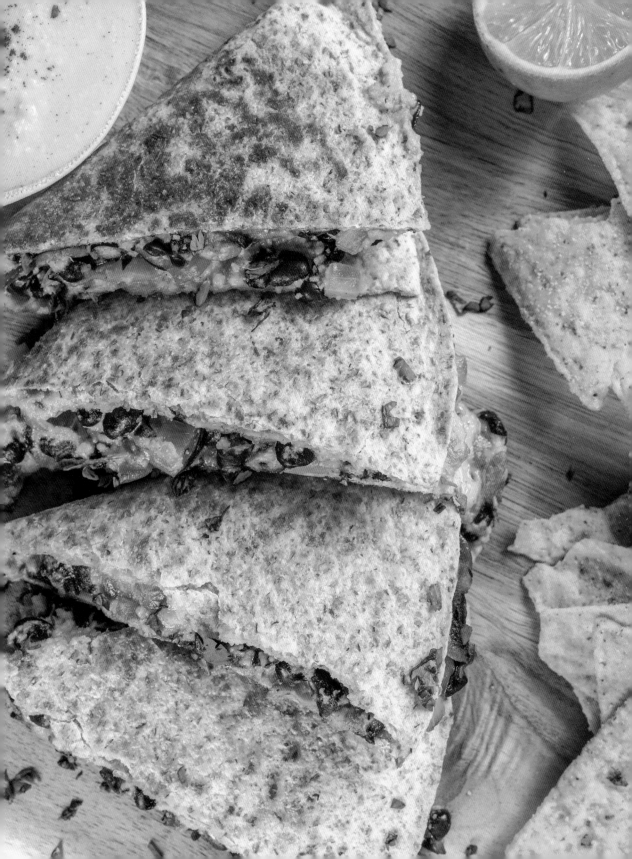

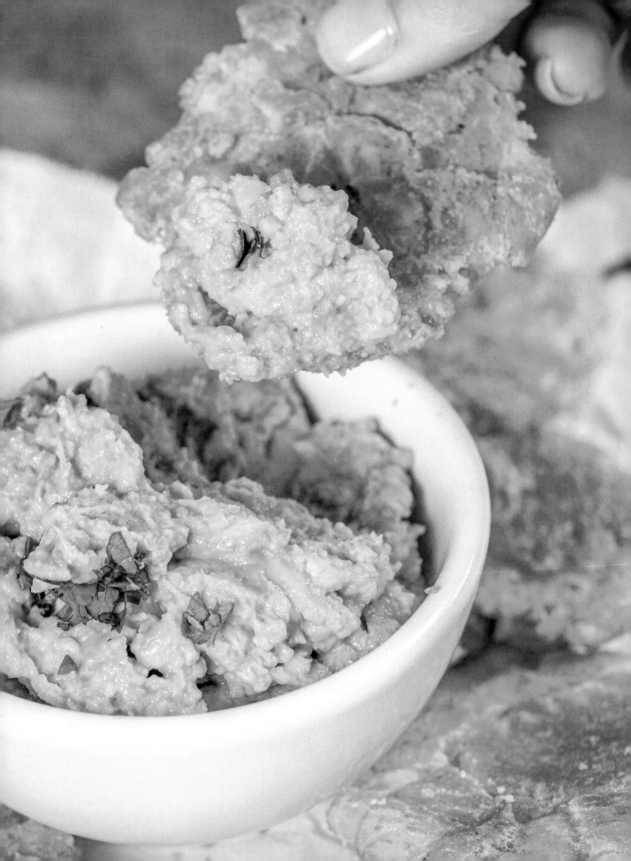

Snacks

Garlic Spiced Edamame

Per serving: Calories: 207 | Fat: 9g | Carbs: 16g | Fiber: 9g | Protein: 21g

1 ½ cups frozen edamame, in the pod

1 tablespoon less-sodium soy sauce or tamari

1 garlic clove, minced

¼ teaspoon paprika

Serves: 1   ◷ Cooking Time: 5 minutes

Curb hunger and satisfy salt cravings with edamame. This great protein-packed, low-carb snack gives you energy without spiking your blood sugar.

NOTES:

Watch the time: You may have to experiment with the cooking time depending on your microwave.

Make it soy-free: Use lima beans in place of the edamame. Swap the soy sauce for coconut aminos.

Save time: Skip the seasonings and just add a pinch of salt!

1. Evenly spread the edamame in a microwave-safe dish and sprinkle 2 tablespoons of water over the top. Cover slightly, allowing room for some air to escape.

2. Cook in the microwave for 2–3 minutes, or until the edamame is steaming and hot.

3. Top with the soy sauce, garlic, and paprika. Toss until combined.

*Nutrition information is per serving

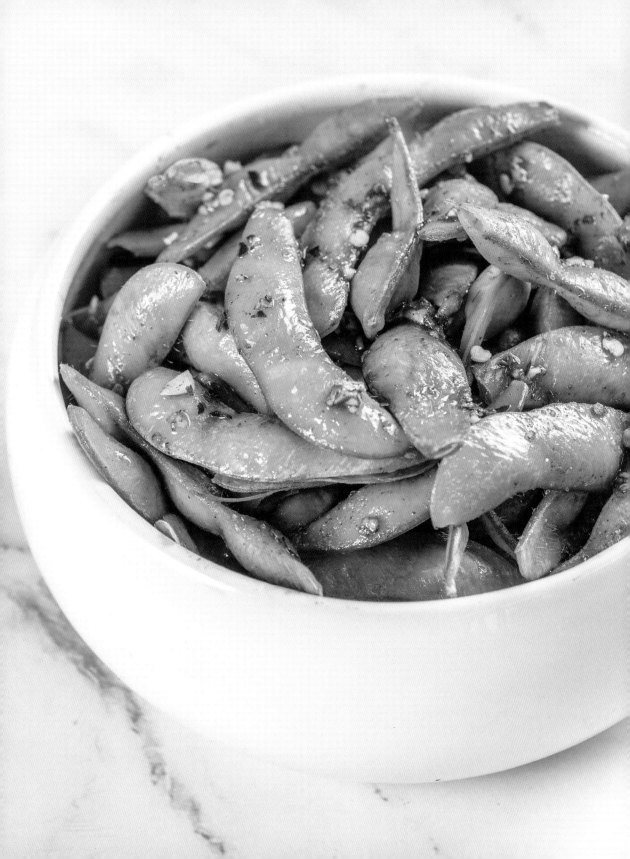

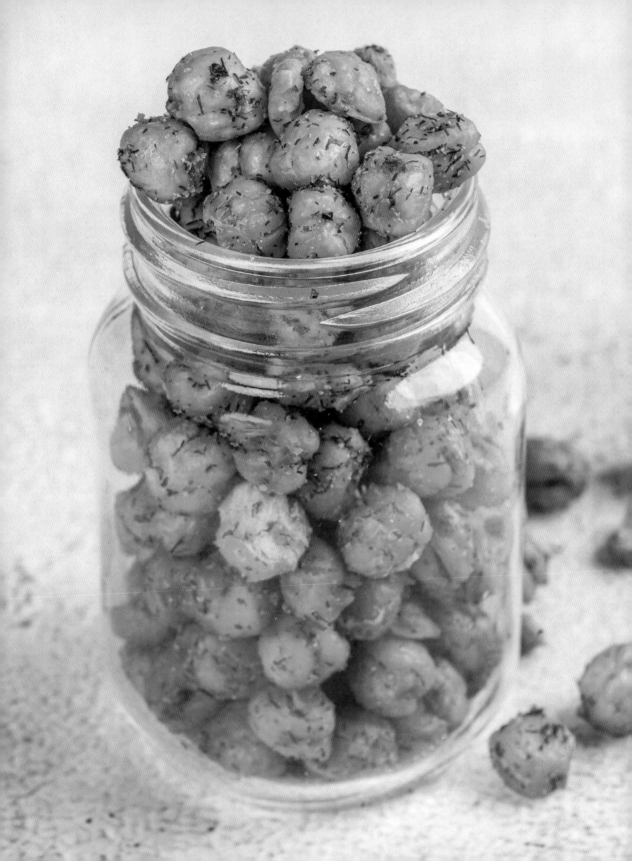

Crispy Chickpeas (3 Ways)

BASE INGREDIENTS

1 (15-ounce) can chickpeas, drained and rinsed

RANCH

½ tablespoon apple cider vinegar

1 teaspoon dried dill

1 teaspoon dried parsley

½ teaspoon garlic powder

½ teaspoon onion powder

½ teaspoon salt

¼ teaspoon black pepper

SALT AND VINEGAR

¼ cup white wine vinegar

1 teaspoon salt

NACHO "CHEESE"

¼ cup nutritional yeast

1 teaspoon paprika

1 teaspoon onion powder

1 teaspoon chili powder

½ teaspoon salt

Serves: 2   **Cooking Time: 45 minutes**

Flavorful and crunchy, these crispy chickpeas satisfy any snack craving. Chickpeas are a great plant-based protein and fiber source—snacking on foods rich in protein and fiber helps maintain energy and keeps blood sugar levels steady throughout the day..

1. Preheat the oven to 375°F and line a baking sheet with parchment paper.

2. For the salt and vinegar variation, soak the chickpeas in white wine vinegar for 30 minutes. Then drain but don't rinse them.

3. Pat the chickpeas dry with a kitchen towel, removing as many of the skins as possible.

4. Spread the chickpeas out in one even layer on the baking sheet and spray with olive oil cooking spray. Bake for 30 minutes.

5. Toss the chickpeas with all the spices and seasonings for your preferred variation, then bake for an additional 10 minutes, watching them closely as they can burn easily.

6. Cool and store in an airtight container at room temperature for up to one week.

Per serving Ranch:
Calories: 210 | Fat: 3g | Carbs: 35g | Fiber: 10g | Protein: 11g

● Carb-to-Fiber Ratio: 3.5:1

Per serving Salt and Vinegar:
Calories: 210 | Fat: 3g | Carbs: 34g | Fiber: 9g | Protein: 11g

● Carb-to-Fiber Ratio: 3:1

Per serving Nacho "Cheese":
Calories: 243 | Fat: 4g | Carbs: 38g | Fiber: 12g | Protein: 15g

● Carb-to-Fiber Ratio: 3:1

*Nutrition information is per serving

Toast (3 Ways)

1 slice whole-grain bread, toasted

Serves: 1   🕐 Cooking Time: 5 minutes

NUT BUTTER AND FRUIT

1 ½ tablespoons nut butter

½ cup berries or 1 apple, sliced

There's no need to fear or limit bread with diabetes. Instead, opt for whole-grain toast, which provides a significant amount of the protein and fiber needed to control blood sugar. Whole-grain bread also comes packed with B vitamins, which aid with carbohydrate metabolism.

HUMMUS AND CUCUMBER

3 tablespoons Oil-Free Hummus (page 226) or store-bought hummus

¼ cucumber, sliced

1. Spread the nut butter, hummus, or mashed avocado on the toast.
2. Top with the remaining ingredients.

AVOCADO AND TOMATO

¼ medium avocado, mashed

¼ cup sliced cherry tomatoes

½ tablespoon hemp seeds

Per slice Nut Butter and Berries toast:
Calories: 247 | Fat: 10g | Carbs: 32g | Fiber: 6g | Protein: 10g

● Carb-to-Fiber Ratio: 5:1

Per slice Hummus and Cucumber toast:
Calories: 227 | Fat: 10g | Carbs: 27g | Fiber: 6g | Protein: 10g

● Carb-to-Fiber Ratio: 4.5:1

Per slice Avocado and Tomato toast:
Calories: 224 | Fat: 12g | Carbs: 24g | Fiber: 7g | Protein: 8g

● Carb-to-Fiber Ratio: 3:1

NOTES:

Make it nut-free: Use sunflower seed butter in place of the nut butter.

Make it gluten-free: Use gluten-free bread, rice cakes, or corn tortillas.

*Nutrition information is per serving

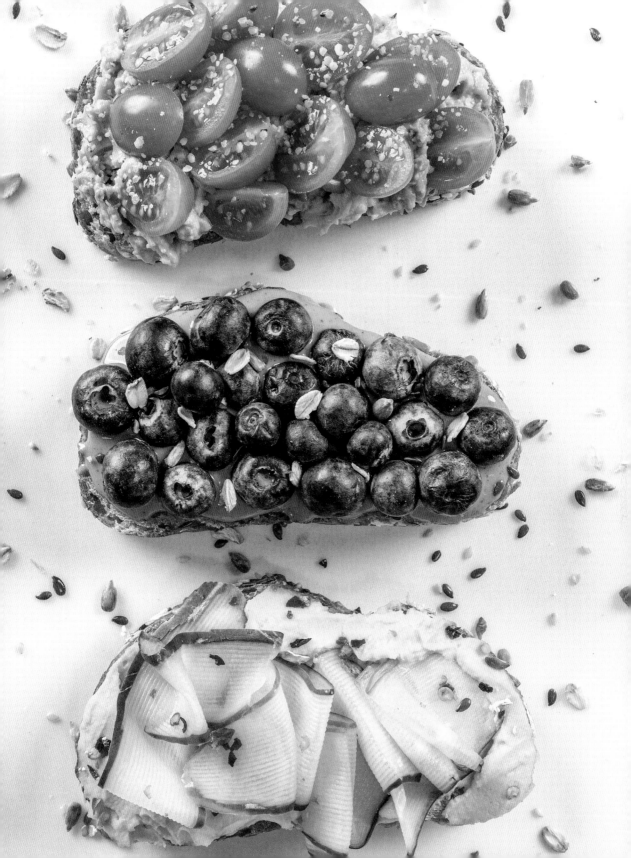

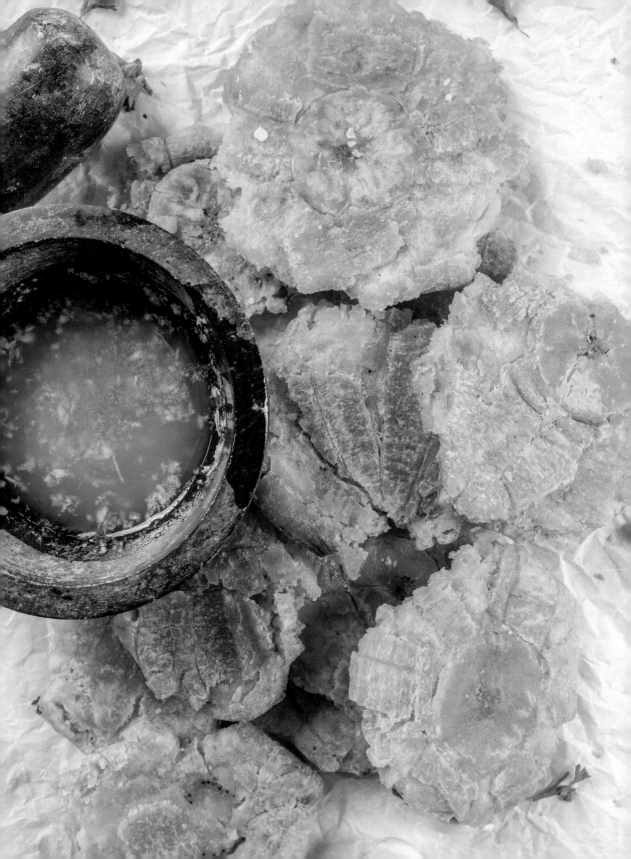

Twice-Air-Fried Tostones with Protein-Packed Guacamole

Per 2-4 tostones and ½ cup guacamole: Calories: 363 | Fat: 15g | Carbs: 59g | Fiber: 11g | Protein: 6g

2 large green plantains

1 teaspoon salt, or more to taste

½ teaspoon garlic powder

1 serving Protein-Packed Guacamole (page 229)

NOTES:

Watch the time: You may have to experiment with the cooking time depending on your air fryer.

No air fryer? Follow the same steps using an oven.

Serves: 4   ⏱ Cooking Time: 35 minutes

Tostones are a common side dish from Latin American and Caribbean cuisine. Air frying them helps cut back on the amount of oil used during preparation. Tostones are made from unripe plantains, which contain resistant starch. This fiber-like starch isn't absorbed in the bloodstream, making it great for managing your blood sugar. Pairing tostones with our protein-packed guacamole helps increase the protein to create a more balanced snack.

1. Preheat the air fryer (if needed) to 350°F. Line a baking sheet with parchment paper.

2. Peel the plantains and cut them into ½-inch diagonal pieces.

3. Spray the plantains lightly with olive oil spray and air fry for 7 minutes on each side.

4. Meanwhile, combine ½ cup water with the salt and garlic powder in a small bowl.

5. Remove the plantains from the air fryer and increase the temperature of the air fryer to 450°F. Press the plantains using a plantain presser, the bottom of a cup, or a mason jar.

6. Bathe each pressed plantain in the water-salt-garlic mixture.

7. Air fry the plantains one more time for 5 minutes on each side, or until crispy and the edges are golden brown.

8. Serve with the protein-packed guacamole.

*Nutrition information is per serving

Red Lentil Cakes

Per 2 lentil cakes: Calories: 152 | Fat: 0g | Carbs: 27g | Fiber: 6g | Protein: 10g

1 cup dried red lentils

1 teaspoon salt

½ teaspoon dried oregano or Italian seasoning

NOTES:

Add veggies: Top with avocado, tomatoes, and any other veggies of your choice for a filling snack.

Makes 9-10   ○ Cooking Time: 15 minutes, plus 3 hours soaking time

Our take on flatbread, these red lentil cakes are chock-full of protein and fiber, two crucial ingredients for a filling and blood sugar-friendly snack.

1. Soak the lentils in 2 cups of water for a minimum of 3 hours, or overnight.

2. Pour the soaked lentils, salt, oregano, and water into a blender and blend until creamy.

3. Preheat a nonstick pan or griddle over medium-high heat.

4. Use a measuring cup to pour in ⅓ cup of batter for each lentil cake. Cook until bubbles pop in the batter, 3–5 minutes, similar to cooking pancakes.

5. Flip and cook on the other side until golden, about 3 minutes. Repeat with the remaining batter.

6. Eat immediately or store in a container in the fridge for up to a week.

*Nutrition information is per serving

Cheesy Popcorn

Per 3½ cups: Calories: 121 | Fat: 1g | Carbs: 20g | Fiber: 5g | Protein: 8g

¼ cup popping corn kernels

2 tablespoons nutritional yeast

1 teaspoon salt

NOTES:

Watch the time: You may have to experiment with the cooking time depending on your microwave.

Serves: 2   🕐 Cooking Time: 15 minutes

Pop some popcorn for a fun, fiber-rich, and blood sugar-friendly snack! Sprinkle with nutritional yeast for a cheesy flavor and nutrient boost, or experiment with other spices and herbs to change up the flavor.

1. Place the popcorn kernels in a large microwave-safe bowl with a lid. Cover partway, enough to keep the kernels in the bowl while allowing for some air to escape.

2. Microwave for 3–5 minutes, or until the popping slows to every 1–2 seconds. Remove the bowl from the microwave.

3. Lightly spray the popcorn with olive oil cooking spray. Add the nutritional yeast and salt and mix well.

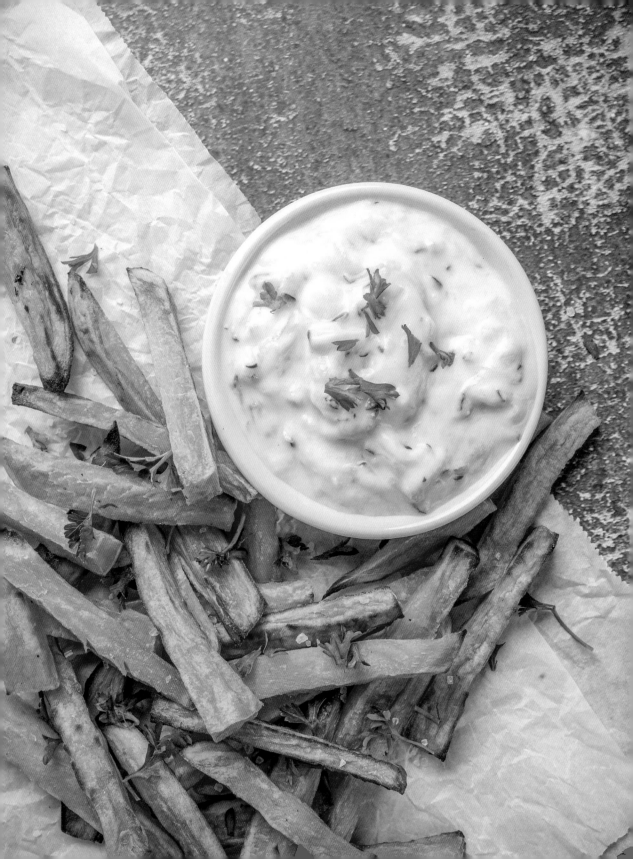

Sweet Potato Fries with Cucumber Yogurt Sauce

Per serving: Calories: 287 | Fat: 6g | Carbs: 56g | Fiber: 9g | Protein: 8g

1 pound sweet potatoes (1 very large or 2 small), peeled

½ teaspoon garlic powder

½ teaspoon paprika

½ teaspoon salt, plus more for sprinkling

¼ teaspoon black pepper

2 tablespoons chopped fresh parsley, for garnish

1 batch Lebanese-Style Cucumber Yogurt Sauce (page 235)

Serves: 2   ⏲ Cooking Time: 40 minutes

Sweet potatoes are full of magnesium, a mineral essential for glucose metabolism. Diets higher in magnesium are associated with a lower risk of type 2 diabetes, and people with insulin resistance appear to have lower magnesium levels. Pair these sweet potato fries with our yogurt sauce to boost the protein content and make this a balanced, filling snack.

1. Preheat the oven to 400°F and line a baking sheet with parchment paper.

2. Cut the sweet potatoes into sticks ¼–½ inch wide and 3 inches long, and spray with olive oil cooking spray.

3. Mix the garlic powder, paprika, salt, and pepper in a small bowl, then toss them with the sweet potatoes.

4. Bake for 15 minutes, or until brown and crisp on the bottom, then flip and cook until the other side is crisp, about 15 minutes.

5. Sprinkle with more salt, garnish with chopped parsley, and serve with the cucumber yogurt sauce.

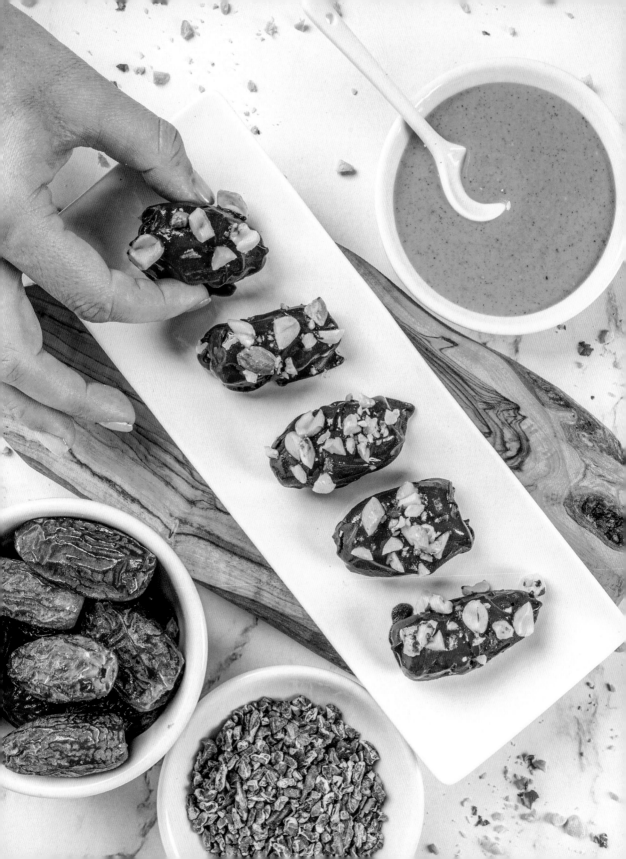

Desserts

No-Sugar-Added Ice Cream (4 Ways)

BASE INGREDIENTS

2 ripe bananas, peeled, sliced, and frozen

CHOCOLATE

3 tablespoons cocoa powder

CREAMY STRAWBERRY

1 cup frozen strawberries

¼ cup unsweetened non-dairy yogurt

PEANUT BUTTER CHOCOLATE

3 tablespoons cocoa powder

2 tablespoons peanut butter

VANILLA CHOCOLATE CHIP

¼ cup no-sugar-added chocolate chips, divided

1 teaspoon vanilla extract

NOTES:

Store leftovers: Freeze in an airtight container for up to three months.

Make it nut-free: Use sunflower seed butter for the peanut butter chocolate version.

Serves: 2   ◷ Cooking Time: 10 minutes

Did you know you can make ice cream from bananas? Our ice cream uses bananas as the base and to add sweetness, so it has no saturated fat and needs no added sugar. Experiment with different fruit and add-ins to create your own favorite varieties.

1. Combine all ingredients in a high-speed blender or food processor. (For the vanilla chocolate chip, add only 2 tablespoons chocolate chips to the blender). Blend, occasionally scraping down the sides, until smooth, 3–5 minutes. For the vanilla chocolate chip, mix in the remaining 2 tablespoons chocolate chips after blending.

2. Scoop into a bowl and enjoy immediately as soft serve, or for firmer ice cream, place in an airtight, freezer-safe container and freeze for at least 1 hour.

Per serving Chocolate:
Calories: 123 | Fat: 2g | Carbs: 32g | Fiber: 6g | Protein: 3g

● Carb-to-Fiber Ratio: 5:1

Per serving Creamy Strawberry:
Calories: 167 | Fat: 2g | Carbs: 39g | Fiber: 6g | Protein: 2g

● Carb-to-Fiber Ratio: 6.5:1

Per serving Peanut Butter Chocolate:
Calories: 219 | Fat: 10g | Carbs: 35g | Fiber: 7g | Protein: 6g

● Carb-to-Fiber Ratio: 5:1

Per serving Vanilla Chocolate Chip:
Calories: 211 | Fat: 8g | Carbs: 43g | Fiber: 13g | Protein: 3g

● Carb-to-Fiber Ratio: 3:1

*Nutrition information is per serving

Chocolate Date Balls

Per 4 date balls: Calories: 154 | Fat: 8g | Carbs: 22g | Fiber: 3g | Protein: 3g

1 cup pitted Medjool dates

¼ cup walnuts or pecans

¼ cup cashews

1 tablespoon cocoa powder

1 tablespoon nut butter or tahini

½ tablespoon unsweetened non-dairy milk

¼ teaspoon vanilla extract

Pinch of salt

Makes 24   🕐 Cooking Time: 30 minutes

These chocolate date balls are a great dessert alternative. Not only are dates great natural sweeteners, but they also contain fiber, keeping the glycemic index low. The lower the glycemic index of a food, the less likely it is to cause a drastic spike in blood sugar.

1. Combine all the ingredients in a food processor and blend until smooth and combined.

2. Roll the mixture into small balls and serve.

NOTES:

Store leftovers: Store chocolate date balls in the refrigerator in an air-tight container for up to ten days or in the freezer for up to four months.

Make it nut-free: Use tahini or sunflower seed butter instead of nut butter. Use sunflower or pumpkin seeds instead of the nuts.

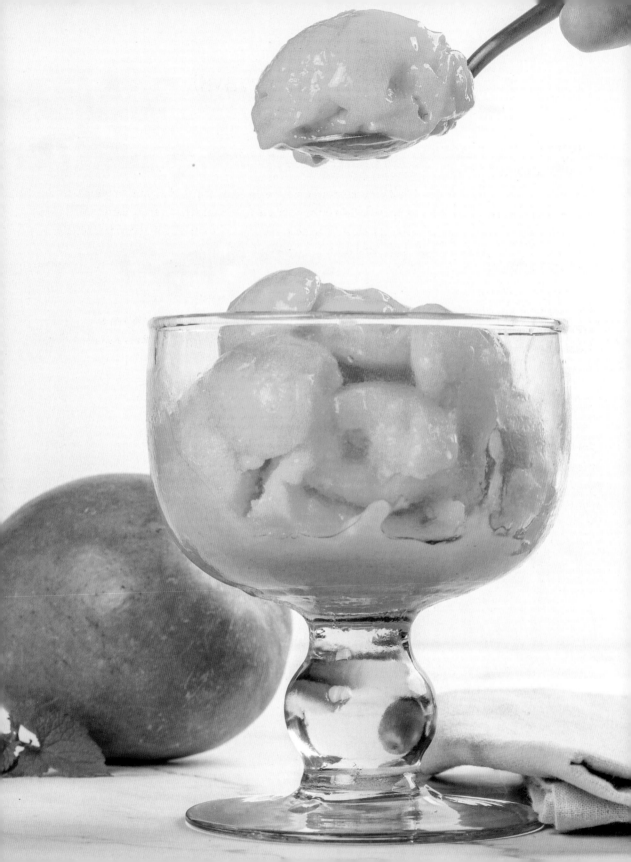

Fruity Sorbet (3 Ways)

CHERRY MINT

2 cups frozen cherries

¼ cup water

2 tablespoons fresh mint

MANGO COCONUT

2 cups frozen mango

½ cup unsweetened coconut yogurt, plain

½ teaspoon ground cinnamon

STRAWBERRY LEMON DATE

2 cups frozen strawberries

3–4 Medjool dates

2 teaspoons fresh lemon juice

¼ cup water

Serves: 2   🕐 Cooking Time: 5 minutes

Fruity sorbets provide a sweet fix along with nutrients and antioxidants important for regulating blood sugar. Adding herbs and spices to the sorbet increases this dessert alternative's antioxidant content and blood sugar benefits.

1. Allow the fruit to thaw for approximately 5 minutes.

2. Combine all the ingredients in a food processor or high-speed blender. Blend until smooth, scraping down the sides as needed to ensure all ingredients are evenly blended.

3. Serve immediately.

Per serving Cherry Mint:
Calories: 72 | Fat: 1g | Carbs: 17g | Fiber: 3g | Protein: 1g

● Carb-to-Fiber Ratio: 6:1

Per serving Mango Coconut:
Calories: 128 | Fat: 2g | Carbs: 28g | Fiber: 4g | Protein: 2g

● Carb-to-Fiber Ratio: 7:1

Per serving Strawberry Lemon Date:
Calories: 168 | Fat: 0g | Carbs: 44g | Fiber: 7g | Protein: 2g

● Carb-to-Fiber Ratio: 6:1

Chocolate-Covered Snicker Dates

Per 2 dates: Calories: 286 | Fat: 14g | Carbs: 49g | Fiber: 14g | Protein: 6g

6 Medjool dates

1 tablespoon peanut butter

2 tablespoons crushed peanuts, divided

6 tablespoons no-sugar-added chocolate chips

NOTES:

Save time: Instead of melting the chocolate, add the chocolate chips inside the dates along with the peanut butter.

Make it nut-free: Use sunflower seed butter and crushed sunflower or pumpkin seeds.

Plan ahead: Make a big batch and store them in the freezer for one to two months.

Serves: 3 🕐 Cooking Time: 20 minutes

Snicker dates are great for a balanced bite-sized dessert or afternoon sweet treat. The fiber in the dates and the protein and healthy fats in the peanut butter help to slow the digestion of the naturally-occurring sugar found in dates.

1. Line a platter with parchment paper.

2. Cut a slit into each date and remove any pits.

3. Fill each date with about ½ teaspoon peanut butter and about 1 teaspoon crushed peanuts. Set aside.

4. Melt the chocolate chips in a double boiler, or in a microwave-safe bowl in the microwave. If using a microwave, melt the chocolate in 15-second increments, stirring between each; 1–2 minutes total.

5. Using a toothpick, dip each date into the melted chocolate and use a spoon to coat the date until completely covered. Place the chocolate-covered dates on the prepared platter. Sprinkle the remaining crushed peanuts on top of each date.

6. Place the dates in the freezer for at least 1-2 hours to allow the chocolate to set.

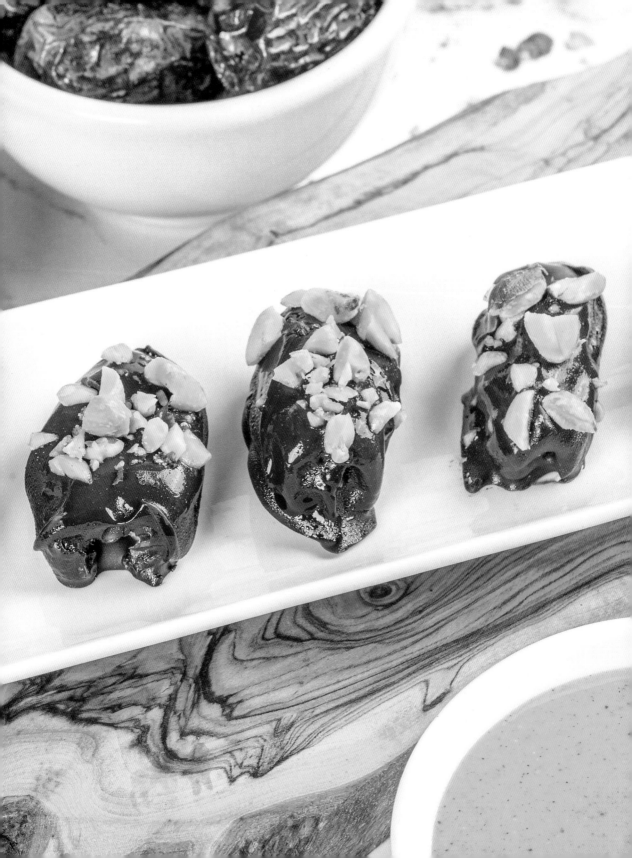

Chocolate Chia Pudding

Per serving: Calories: 166 | Fat: 10g | Carbs: 14g | Fiber: 10g | Protein: 8g

1 cup unsweetened non-dairy milk

1 ½ tablespoons 100% cocoa powder

1–2 tablespoons monk
fruit sweetener

½ teaspoon vanilla extract

¼ cup chia seeds

Serves: 2

🕐 Cooking Time: 10 minutes,
plus 4 hours soaking time

Chia seed pudding makes for a decadent and filling dessert. Moreover, chia seeds are an excellent source of healthy fats and fiber. Adding chia seeds to the diet can help improve insulin resistance.

1. Combine the milk, cocoa powder, monk fruit sweetener, and vanilla extract in a bowl and whisk until combined.

2. Add the chia seeds and stir. Let sit for 5 minutes, then stir again.

3. Refrigerate the mixture for at least 4 hours.

4. When ready to serve, stir to mix the pudding.

NOTES:

Add more flavor: Top with your favorite fresh berries.

No monk fruit sweetener? Use 1–2 chopped dates instead.

*Nutrition information is per serving

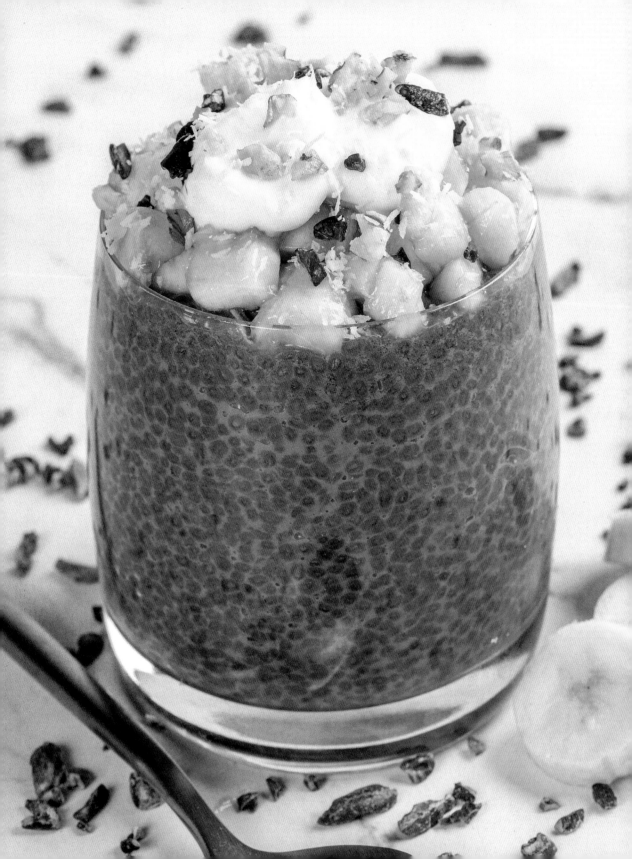

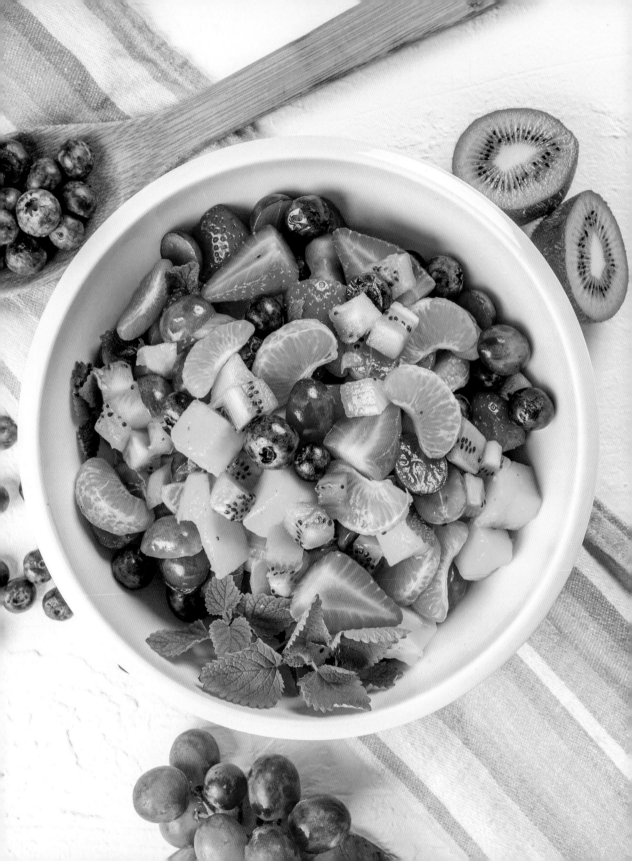

Epic Rainbow Fruit Salad

Per 1 cup: Calories: 100 | Fat: 1g | Carbs: 25g | Fiber: 4g | Protein: 2g

1 cup cubed mango

1 cup halved strawberries, stems removed

1 cup blueberries

1 cup halved red grapes

3 kiwis, peeled and chopped

2 mandarins, peeled and separated into segments

¼ cup fresh mint

Juice of ½ lime

Serves: 6   🕐 Cooking Time: 15 minutes

Fruit is an excellent source of antioxidants, which minimize cellular damage that results from stress, such as high blood sugar and diabetes. And diets high in fruit—like a plant-based diet—are associated with lower risks of developing type 2 diabetes.

1. Combine the mango, strawberries, blueberries, grapes, kiwi, and mandarin slices in a large bowl.
2. Add the mint and lime. Mix and enjoy.

NOTES:

Change it up: Use watermelon, peach, or pineapple.

Save time: Buy precut fruit.

Reduce food waste: Freeze extra fruit and use it for smoothies or sorbets. Use leftover mint for No-Sugar-Added Berry Chia Jam (page 238).

Slow Cooker Cinnamon Applesauce

Per ⅔ cup: Calories: 95 | Fat: 0g | Carbs: 25g | Fiber: 6g | Protein: 0g

6 large apples, cored and diced

2 cinnamon sticks

Serves: 6   ◷ Cooking Time: 15 minutes, plus 4 hours in the slow cooker

NOTES:

Store leftovers: **Refrigerate in an airtight container for up to ten days, or freeze for up to a year.**

Many applesauces contain added sugar. But this is unnecessary, as cooking caramelizes the sugar from apples, making a naturally sweet applesauce. Leaving the skins on the apples provides additional nutritional benefits: the skins are rich in polyphenols (molecules in plant-based foods with health benefits). Eating polyphenol-rich foods is associated with a lower risk of type 2 diabetes and improved blood glucose levels and insulin sensitivity.

1. Combine the chopped apple, cinnamon, and ½ cup water in a slow cooker and stir well to mix.

2. Cook on high for 4 hours, stirring occasionally.

3. Remove the cinnamon sticks. Use an immersion blender to puree the applesauce, or transfer to a blender and puree to your preferred consistency.

*Nutrition information is per serving

Grilled Peaches with Cinnamon

Per serving: Calories: 62 | Fat: 0g | Carbs: 15g | Fiber: 3g | Protein: 1g

1 peach, sliced in half with
pit removed

Olive oil, for brushing

½ teaspoon ground cinnamon

Serves: 1   ◷ Cooking Time: 15 minutes

Peaches are a good source of vitamin C, which acts as an antioxidant
in the body to reduce the cellular damage that can occur with high
blood sugar.

NOTES:

Store leftovers: Refrigerate in an
airtight container for up to four
days. To prevent browning, squeeze
lemon juice over the peaches
before refrigerating.

Add additional toppings: Top with
non-dairy yogurt, shredded coconut,
or hemp seeds.

1. Preheat a grill or grill pan to medium heat.

2. Brush the peach halves with a little olive oil to prevent them from
sticking to the grill.

3. Place the peaches cut side down on the grill. Grill until soft and
toasted, about 4 minutes per side. Remove from the heat.

4. Sprinkle the sliced peaches with the cinnamon. Serve immediately.

Fudgy Brownies

Per brownie: Calories: 171 | Fat: 10g | Carbs: 16g | Fiber: 4g | Protein: 5g

3 large, ripe bananas

½ cup peanut butter

½ cup 100% cocoa powder

1 teaspoon baking powder

Pinch of salt

Makes 8

🕐 Cooking Time: 45 minutes

Fudgier than a classic brownie, this version uses cocoa powder for its chocolate flavor. Cocoa is rich in polyphenols, compounds in plant-based foods that benefit health. In particular, the polyphenols in cocoa may help reduce insulin resistance.

NOTES:

Make it nut-free: Use sunflower seed butter in place of the peanut butter.

More sweetness? Add 2-3 chopped dates.

1. Preheat the oven to 350°F. Line an 8x8-inch brownie pan with parchment paper.

2. Mash the bananas in a bowl. Add the remaining ingredients and mix until well combined.

3. Transfer the mixture to the brownie pan and bake for 25–30 minutes, until the brownies are set.

4. Let cool for 10 minutes to solidify, then cut into 8 squares for serving.

*Nutrition information is per serving

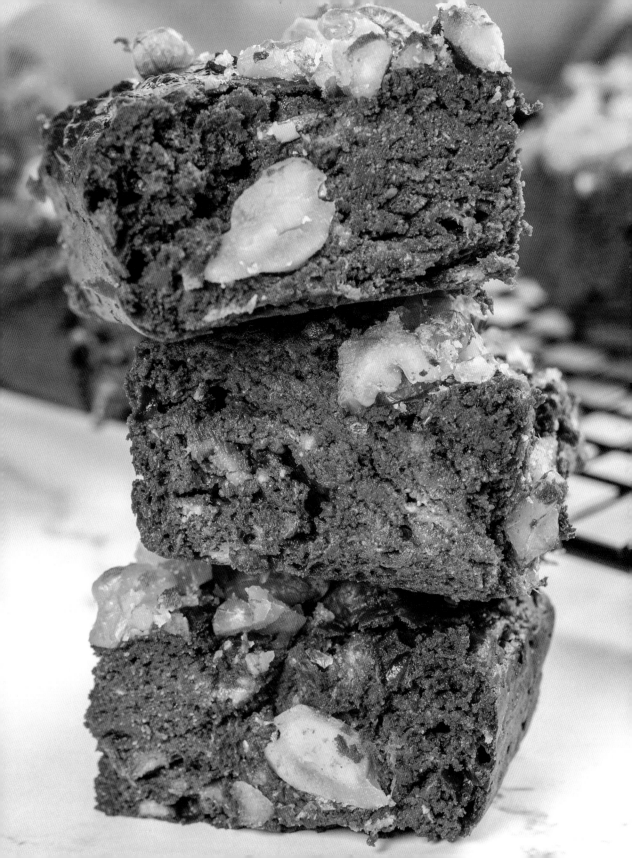

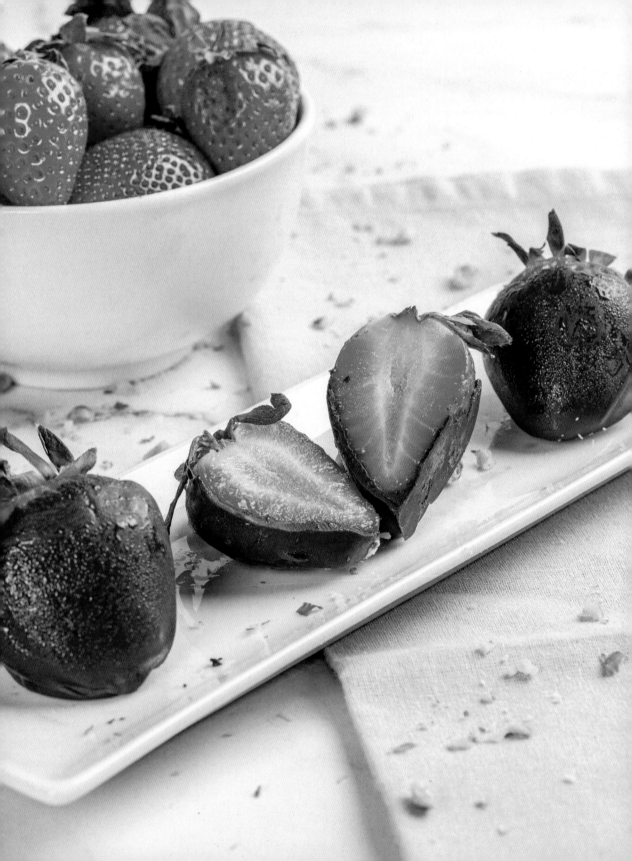

Chocolate-Covered Strawberries

Per 3 strawberries: Calories: 158 | Fat: 11g | Carbs: 27g | Fiber: 15g | Protein: 3g

½ cup no-sugar-added chocolate chips

½ pound strawberries (5–10)

Serves: 3   🕐 Cooking Time: 20 minutes, plus 1 hour chilling time

You can still enjoy chocolate while monitoring your blood sugar. Opt for dark chocolate or one without added sugar to maintain optimal blood glucose. Pairing the chocolate with fruit—such as the strawberries in this recipe—keeps the dessert healthy and balanced.

1. Line a baking sheet with parchment paper.

2. Melt the chocolate chips in a double boiler or in a microwave-safe bowl in the microwave. If using a microwave, melt the chocolate in 15-second increments, stirring between each; 1–2 minutes total.

3. Dip strawberries into the melted chocolate. Let excess chocolate drip off the strawberries before placing them on the baking sheet.

4. Once all of the strawberries are coated in chocolate, place the baking sheet in the refrigerator for at least 1 hour to let the chocolate harden before serving.

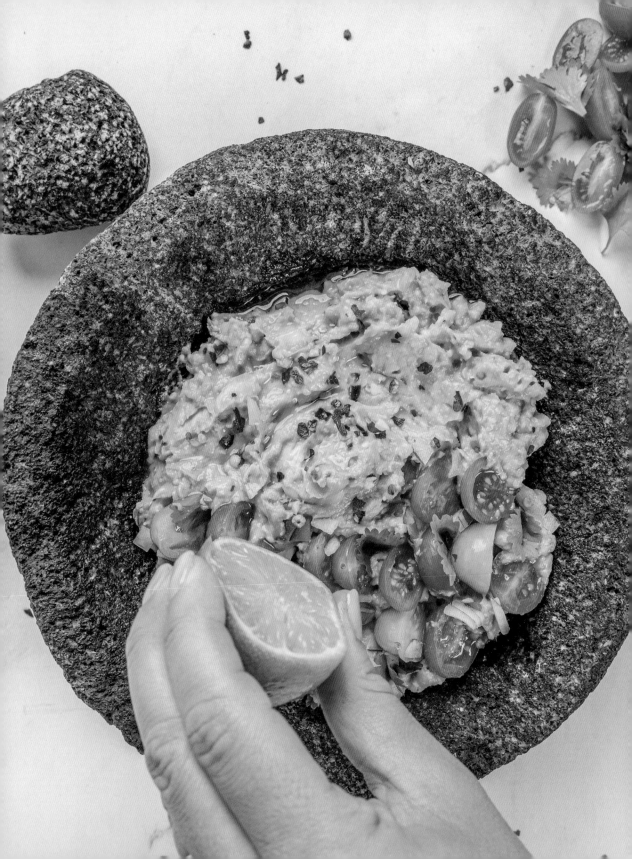

Sauces, Dips, and Dressings

Lentil "No Meat" Sauce

Per 1 cup: Calories: 198 | Fat: 10g | Carbs: 22g | Fiber: 7g | Protein: 8g

½ large onion, diced

3 garlic cloves, roughly chopped

¾ cup small-diced carrots

1 teaspoon dried oregano

¾ teaspoon salt

¼ teaspoon black pepper

⅛ teaspoon red pepper flakes

⅛ teaspoon ground cumin

2 tablespoons plus 2 teaspoons tomato paste

2 medium tomatoes, diced with juices reserved

2 cups vegetable stock, plus more for sautéing

⅔ cup dried red lentils

6 tablespoons crushed walnuts

NOTES:

Make it nut-free: Use hemp seeds instead of walnuts.

Serve it up: Serve over whole-wheat, or bean pasta, or zucchini noodles.

Store leftovers: Store sauce in an airtight container in the fridge for up to five days.

Serves: 3   🕐 Cooking Time: 35 minutes

This no-meat sauce contains a surprise ingredient—walnuts. Walnuts are a great plant-based source of omega-3 fatty acids, a type of poly-unsaturated fat beneficial for health. In particular, omega-3 fatty acids contribute to lower levels of inflammation, which is common with type 2 diabetes. What's more, regular consumption of walnuts is associated with a lower risk of diabetes due to the high fiber and protein content found in this type of nut.

1. In a large skillet over medium heat, sauté the onion and garlic in a splash of vegetable stock for 2–3 minutes, adding more vegetable stock as needed.

2. Add the carrots, oregano, salt, pepper, red pepper flakes, and cumin. Cook for 7–8 minutes, stirring occasionally, adding more vegetable stock as needed to prevent sticking.

3. Add the tomato paste and tomatoes and their juices and cook for 2–3 minutes.

4. Add the vegetable stock, lentils, and walnuts. Bring to a boil, then cover tightly, lower the heat to low, and simmer gently for 20–25 minutes, or until the lentils are tender. Uncover.

5. Continue cooking uncovered until most of the liquid has cooked off, or until desired consistency is reached.

*Nutrition information is per serving

Herbed "Ricotta" Filling

Per ½ cup: Calories: 75 | Fat: 4g | Carbs: 4g | Fiber: 2g | Protein: 9g

½ small yellow onion, roughly chopped

4 garlic cloves, roughly chopped

½ teaspoon dried oregano or Italian seasoning

1 teaspoon salt

¼ teaspoon black pepper

1 (14-ounce) block tofu, extra firm, drained and pressed

1 cup spinach, roughly chopped

2 tablespoons nutritional yeast

2 tablespoons fresh lemon juice

NOTES:

Make it soy-free: Use 2 cups of raw cashews in place of the tofu. You may need to add water to achieve the desired thickness.

Store leftovers: Refrigerate in an airtight container for up to five days.

Makes 3 cups   ◷ Cooking Time: 15 minutes

Blend tofu to make a smooth, creamy texture similar to ricotta cheese. Adding onion and spinach creates a more substantial filling for use in any recipe that calls for ricotta, such as lasagna or eggplant roll-ups. Moreover, using tofu in place of ricotta enhances the protein and reduces the fat content of your dish.

1. In nonstick pan (or a pan lightly sprayed with olive oil cooking spray), combine the onions and garlic over medium heat. Add the oregano or Italian seasoning, salt, and pepper and sauté for 3–5 minutes, or until the onions are translucent. Allow the mixture to cool.

2. Break up the tofu and transfer it to a food processor or a high-speed blender.

3. Add all the remaining ingredients, including the onion and garlic mixture, and blend until just combined.

*Nutrition information is per serving

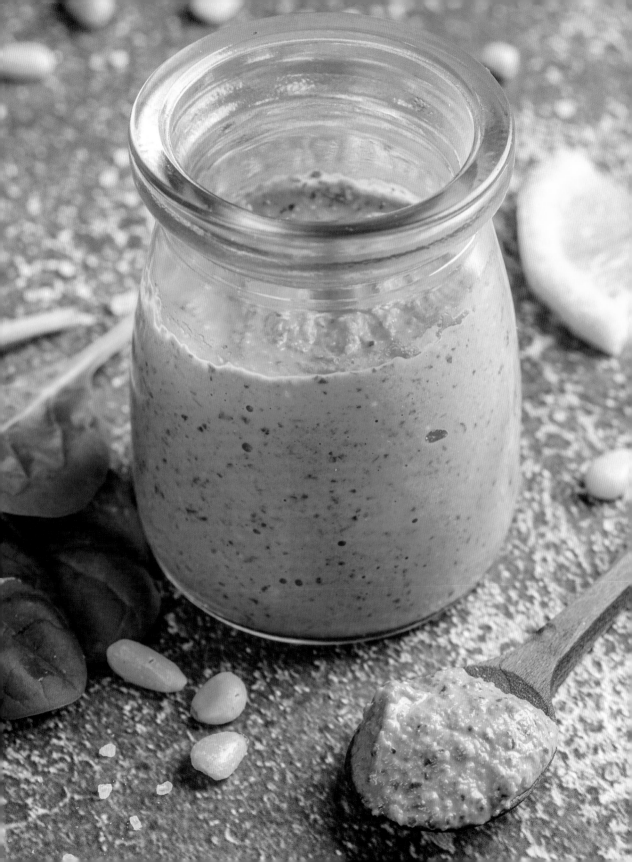

Basil Spinach Pesto

Per ¼ cup: Calories: 172 | Fat: 16g | Carbs: 6g | Fiber: 2g | Protein: 5g

2 cups fresh basil leaves (stems removed)

2 cups fresh baby spinach

1 medium tomato, roughly chopped

1 cup raw pine nuts

¼ cup nutritional yeast

2 garlic cloves

½ teaspoon salt

Black pepper, to taste

1 tablespoon fresh lemon juice

Makes 1½ cups   🕐 Cooking Time: 5 minutes

Our oil-free pesto packs extra vegetables—spinach and tomatoes—to boost its nutritional and fiber content. The touch of nutritional yeast mimics the Parmesan cheese typically found in pesto, but without the saturated fat.

1. In a high-speed blender or food processor, blend all the ingredients except the lemon juice until the mixture is smooth.

2. Scrape down the sides, add the lemon juice, and blend again.

NOTES:

No pine nuts? Use sunflower seeds or cashews.

Store leftovers: Refrigerate in an airtight container for up to five days.

Fresh Basil Tomato Sauce

Per ½ cup: Calories: 37 | Fat: 0g | Carbs: 8g | Fiber: 2g | Protein: 2g

6–8 medium tomatoes

½ yellow onion, diced

6 garlic gloves, minced

3 tablespoons chopped fresh basil

1 tablespoon monk fruit sweetener

1 tablespoon olive oil, optional

½ tablespoon dried oregano

2 teaspoons tomato paste

1 teaspoon salt

¼ teaspoon black pepper

NOTES:

Store leftovers: Refrigerate in an airtight container for up to five days or freeze in an airtight container for three to four months.

Makes 2½ cups 🕐 Cooking Time: 20 minutes

You would be surprised to learn that many store-bought tomato sauces contain added sugar. This homemade version uses a small amount of monk fruit to balance the acidity of the tomatoes, but feel free to leave it out if your sauce tastes sweet enough.

1. Bring a large pot of water to a boil. Add the tomatoes and let boil for 10 minutes, or until the skin starts to peel off.

2. Meanwhile, in a nonstick skillet (or a skillet lightly sprayed with olive oil cooking spray), sauté the onions and garlic over medium heat for 3–5 minutes, or until the onions become translucent. Set aside.

3. Drain the tomatoes and peel off their skins. Transfer the tomatoes to a blender and blend until smooth.

4. In a saucepan, combine the blended tomatoes with the onions and garlic and all the remaining ingredients over medium-low heat. Stir until combined and heated through.

*Nutrition information is per serving

Cauliflower "Alfredo" Sauce

Per ½ cup: Calories: 56 | Fat: 1g | Carbs: 7g | Fiber: 3g | Protein: 4g

½ head cauliflower, broken into florets (about 3 cups)

½ yellow or white onion, chopped

3 garlic cloves, minced

1 cup unsweetened non-dairy milk

2 tablespoons nutritional yeast

1 teaspoon Dijon mustard

1 teaspoon fresh lemon juice

1 teaspoon salt

½ teaspoon black pepper

NOTES:

Serve it up: Serve over whole-wheat or bean pasta with mushrooms and asparagus.

Store leftovers: Refrigerate in an airtight container for up to five days.

Makes 2 cups   🕐 Cooking Time: 15 minutes

Unlike a typical Alfredo sauce, our version contains no dairy and instead uses a secret ingredient—cauliflower. Blending cauliflower with spices creates a decadent sauce as flavorful and creamy as the classic Alfredo. Bonus: the cauliflower provides a sneaky serving of vegetables and fiber.

1. Bring a pot of water to boil and add the cauliflower. Boil until it is fork-tender, about 10 minutes.

2. Meanwhile, in a nonstick skillet (or a skillet lightly sprayed with olive oil cooking spray), sauté the onion and garlic for 3–5 minutes over medium heat.

3. In a high-speed blender or food processor, combine the cauliflower, onion-garlic mixture, and all remaining ingredients and blend until well combined.

*Nutrition information is per serving

Oil-Free Hummus (6 Ways)

ORIGINAL

1 (15-ounce) can chickpeas, drained and rinsed

⅓ cup tahini

3 tablespoons fresh lemon juice

2 garlic cloves (skip for Roasted Garlic variation)

½ teaspoon salt, or to taste

Black pepper, to taste

¼ cup vegetable stock, or more for a smoother, thinner texture

SPINACH AND ARTICHOKE

2 cups fresh spinach

1 (15-ounce) can artichoke hearts, drained and rinsed

SUN-DRIED TOMATO

¼ cup sun-dried tomatoes

¼ cup chopped fresh basil

ROASTED RED PEPPER

1 roasted red pepper (if from a can, rinse and pat dry)

½ teaspoon smoked paprika

BEET

2 small beets, peeled and roasted

ROASTED GARLIC

1 head of roasted garlic

Makes 1½-2 cups   🕐 Cooking Time: 10 Minutes

Tahini is a sesame-based condiment used in hummus to add smoothness and creaminess. Tahini is also a healthy fat, which improves insulin sensitivity. The high fiber content of hummus—which is rich in tahini and chickpeas—contributes even more to balanced blood sugar!

1. Blend the chickpeas in a food processor until pureed.

2. Add the tahini, lemon juice, garlic, salt, and pepper. Turn the food processor on high and slowly stream in the vegetable stock.

3. Add all the remaining ingredients for your preferred variation. Continue to blend until smooth and creamy.

Per ¼ cup Original:
Calories:161 | Fat: 8g | Carbs: 17g | Fiber: 5g | Protein: 7g

● Carb-to-Fiber Ratio: 3:1

Per ¼ cup Spinach and Artichoke:
Calories: 178 | Fat: 8g | Carbs: 20g | Fiber: 8g | Protein: 8g

● Carb-to-Fiber Ratio: 2.5:1

Per ¼ cup Sun-Dried Tomato:
Calories: 168 | Fat: 9g | Carbs: 18g | Fiber: 5g | Protein: 7g

● Carb-to-Fiber Ratio: 4:1

Per ¼ cup Roasted Red Pepper:
Calories: 166 | Fat: 8g | Carbs: 18g | Fiber: 5g | Protein: 7g

● Carb-to-Fiber Ratio: 4:1

Per ¼ cup Beet:
Calories: 173 | Fat: 8g | Carbs: 19g | Fiber: 6g | Protein: 7g

● Carb-to-Fiber Ratio: 3:1

Per ¼ cup Roasted Garlic:
Calories: 169 | Fat: 8g | Carbs: 19g | Fiber: 5g | Protein: 7g

● Carb-to-Fiber Ratio: 4:1

*Nutrition information is per serving

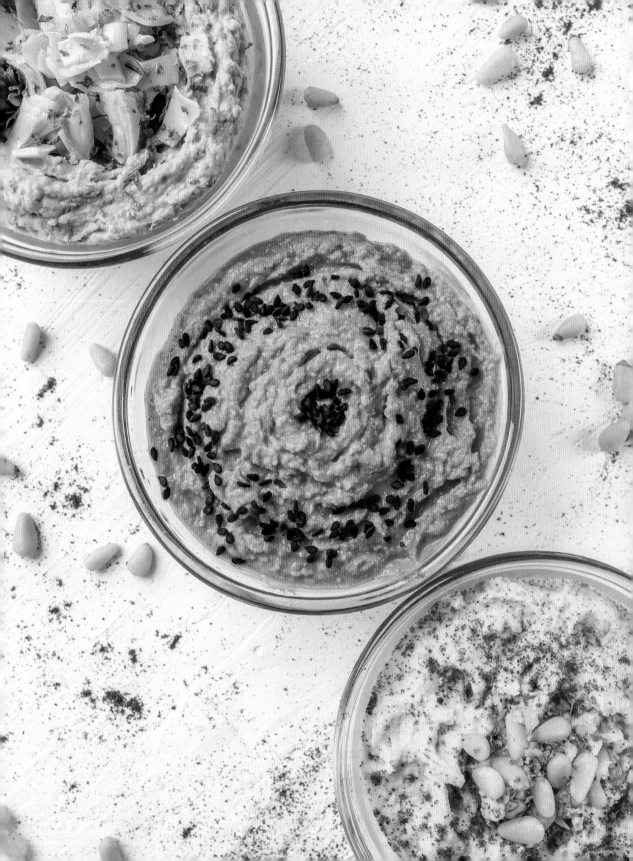

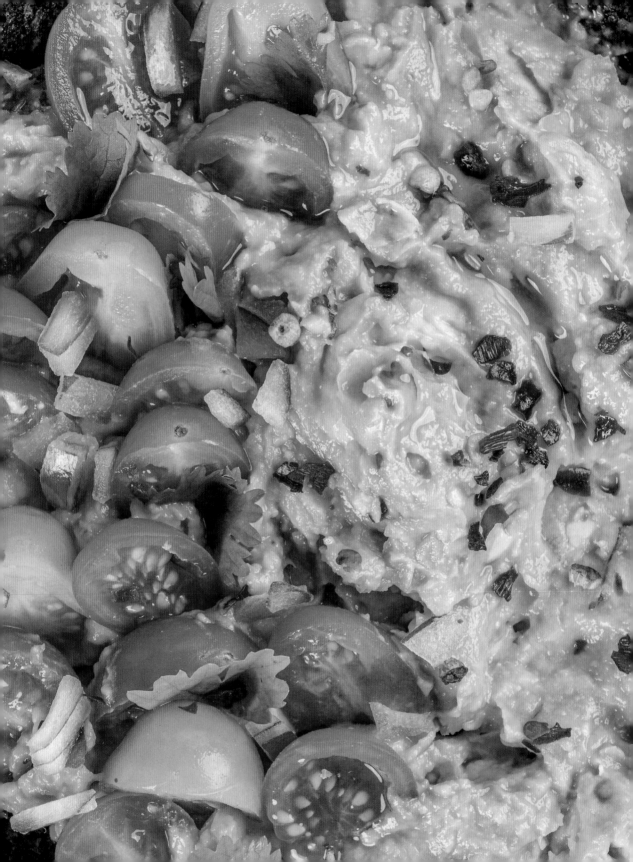

Protein-Packed Guacamole

Per ½ cup: Calories: 201 | Fat: 15g | Carbs: 16g | Fiber: 9g | Protein: 4g

½ cup cooked white beans

2 ripe medium avocados

2 cloves garlic, minced

¼ cup chopped fresh cilantro

¼ cup finely diced white onion

¼ cup chopped tomatoes

2 teaspoons fresh lime juice

½ teaspoon salt

¼ teaspoon red pepper flakes

Black pepper, to taste

NOTES:

Store leftovers: Refrigerate in an airtight container for up three days.

Makes 2 cups   🕐 Cooking Time: 10 minutes

We boosted the protein content in this guacamole with white beans. White beans are a great plant-based source of zinc, a mineral essential for health. In particular, zinc influences insulin functioning, so getting enough zinc can benefit insulin resistance and fasting blood glucose levels.

1. In a medium bowl, mash the white beans with a fork until smooth.

2. Add the avocados and garlic. Mash with a fork again until chunky.

3. Fold in the cilantro, onions, tomatoes, and lime juice.

4. Season with the salt, red pepper flakes, and black pepper. Taste and adjusting the seasoning as needed.

Vitamin C–Rich Mango Salsa

Per ½ cup: Calories: 93 | Fat: 1g | Carbs: 22g | Fiber: 3g | Protein: 2g

1 mango, peeled and diced

1 cup corn, frozen or canned

½ red bell pepper, finely chopped

¼ cup chopped fresh cilantro

2 tablespoons finely chopped red onion

Juice of 1 lime

½ teaspoon salt

NOTES:

Save time: Buy precut mango.

Store leftovers: Refrigerate in an airtight container for up to five days.

Serves: 6   ○ Cooking Time: 10 minutes

This salsa is packed with vitamin C from red pepper, mango, and lime juice. Vitamin C is an antioxidant, so it helps reduce cellular damage in the body that can result from elevated blood sugar levels. Top any dish with some mango salsa for an extra serving of fruit and a vitamin C boost!

1. Combine all the ingredients in a large bowl. Refrigerate until ready to serve.

*Nutrition information is per serving

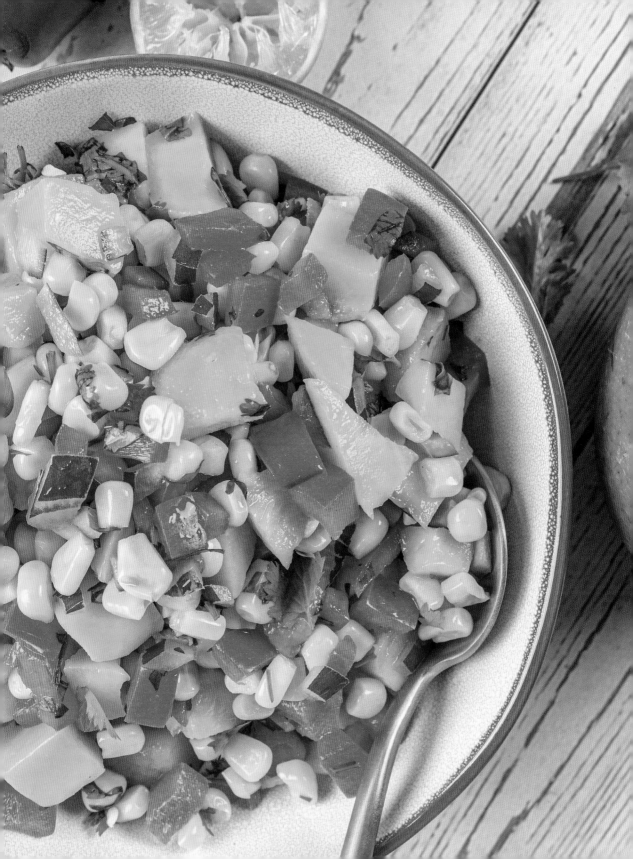

Cashew Nacho "Cheese" Sauce

Per 3 tablespoons: Calories: 153 | Fat: 12g | Carbs: 10g | Fiber: 2g | Protein: 5g

1½ cups raw cashews

1½ cups vegetable stock

¼ cup nutritional yeast

1 tablespoon + 1 teaspoon fresh lemon juice

1 teaspoon onion powder

1 teaspoon garlic powder

1 teaspoon Dijon mustard

½ teaspoon paprika

Pinch of salt

Makes 1⅔ cups   🕐 Cooking Time: 5 minutes

This sauce uses cashews as the base to provide an alternative to regular nacho cheese that is low in saturated fat, but still creamy and full of flavor. Nutritional yeast is a plant-based powder packed with vitamins and minerals that provides a cheesy flavor, and may also benefit blood sugar.

1. In a high-speed blender or food processor, blend all the ingredients together until smooth, scraping down the sides as needed.

NOTES:

Make it nut-free: Use sunflower or pumpkin seeds instead of cashews. You may need to add more vegetable stock to achieve the desired consistency.

Store leftovers: Refrigerate in an airtight container for up to five days.

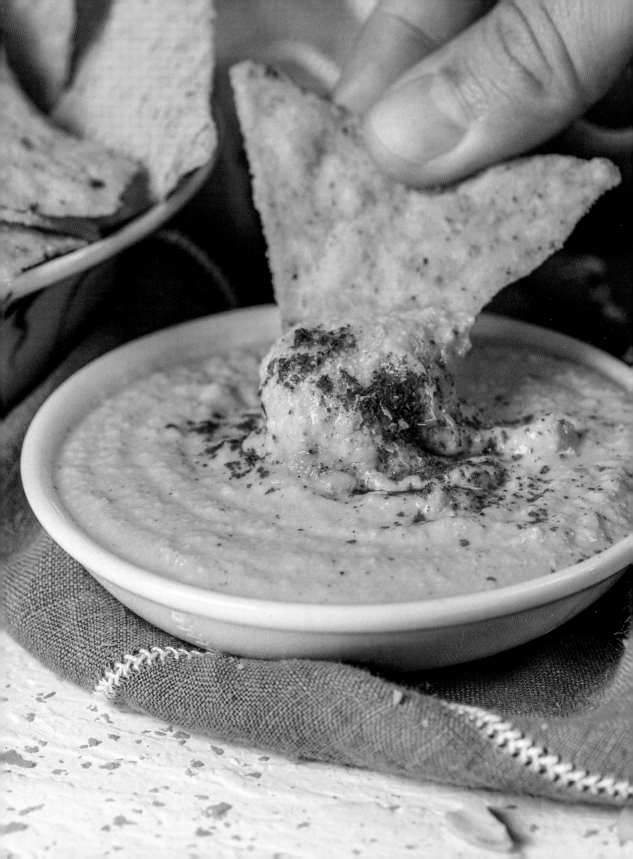

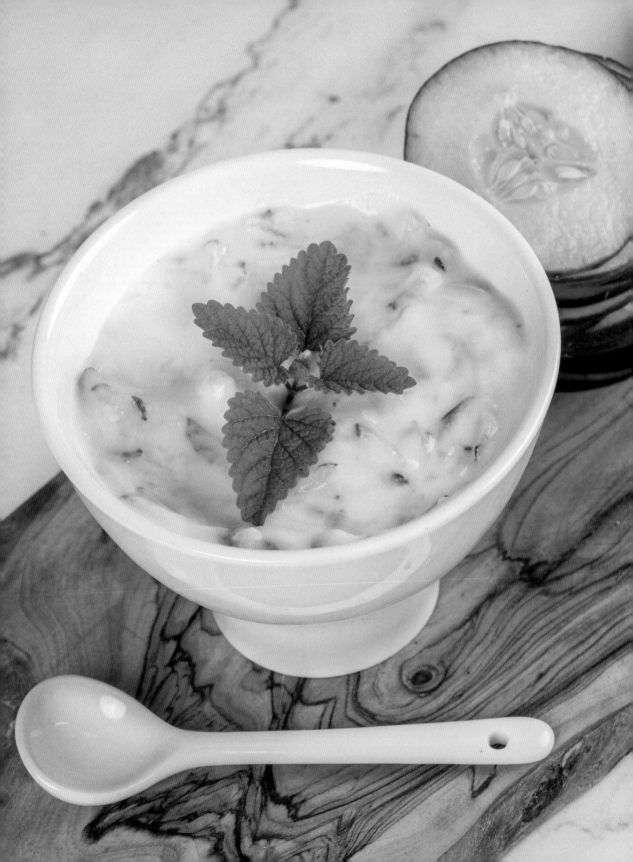

Lebanese-Style Cucumber Yogurt Sauce

Per ½ cup: Calories: 89 | Fat: 5g | Carbs: 9g | Fiber: 2g | Protein: 3g

½ large cucumber, grated

¾ cup unsweetened non-dairy yogurt

Juice of ½ lemon

2 garlic cloves, minced

¼ teaspoon salt

1 teaspoon dried mint or 1 tablespoon chopped fresh mint

NOTES:

Shop smart: Almond- or soy-based yogurt work best for this recipe.

Store leftovers: Refrigerate in an airtight container for up to five days.

Serves: 2   ⏱ Cooking Time: 10 minutes

This Lebanese sauce resembles tzatziki and is made of yogurt, cucumbers, lemon, and garlic. It has a tangy, bright taste and can be used as a dip or a dressing. Ours maintains the integrity of the classic version, but uses non-dairy yogurt to make it plant-based.

1. Wrap the grated cucumber in a paper towel or cheesecloth and squeeze to strain out the excess water.

2. In a bowl, combine the cucumber with all the remaining ingredients and mix until combined.

Peanut Dipping Sauce

Per 2 tablespoons: Calories: 133 | Fat: 11g | Carbs: 6g | Fiber: 1g | Protein: 5g

½ cup creamy peanut butter

3 tablespoons lime juice

2 tablespoons less-sodium soy sauce
or tamari

1–2 tablespoons monk fruit
sweetener, depending on desired
level of sweetness

¼ teaspoon red pepper flakes

NOTES:

Make it nut-free: Use sunflower seed
butter instead of peanut butter.

Store leftovers: Refrigerate in an
airtight container for up to a week.

Make is soy-free: use coconut
aminos in place of the soy sauce.

Makes ¾ cup   ◷ Cooking Time: 5 minutes

This peanut dipping sauce uses monk fruit sweetener instead of sugar
to provide some sweetness, making it more suitable than store-bought
versions for blood sugar management.

1. In a high-speed blender or food processor, combine all of the
ingredients with ¼ cup or more of water to thin out the dressing to
your preferred consistency. Blend until smooth, scraping down the
sides as needed.

*Nutrition information is per serving

Nutty "Cheese" Topper

Per 2 tablespoons: Calories: 80 | Fat: 7g | Carbs: 2g | Fiber: 1g | Protein: 2g

½ cup Brazil nuts

1 tablespoon nutritional yeast

½ teaspoon garlic powder

¼ teaspoon salt

NOTES:

No Brazil nuts? Use raw almonds or cashews instead.

Store leftovers: Refrigerate in an airtight container for up to ten days.

Make it nut-free: Use sunflower or pumpkin seeds in place of the Brazil nuts.

Makes ¾ cup   ○ Cooking Time: 5 minutes

Blending nuts, nutritional yeast, and garlic powder creates a Parmesan-style "cheese" favorable for blood sugar management. Brazil nuts are a rich source of selenium, a nutrient that plays a role in glucose metabolism and fighting stress in the body. Through its antioxidant capacities, selenium may reduce cellular damage, which correlates with insulin resistance. Therefore, including sources of selenium in the diet may help improve insulin resistance.

1. In a high-speed blender or food processor, blend all the ingredients until the mixture reaches the texture of a fine meal.

*Nutrition information is per serving

No-Sugar-Added Berry Chia Jam

Per 2 tablespoons: Calories: 26 | Fat: 1g | Carbs: 7g | Fiber: 2g | Protein: 1g

2 cups frozen strawberries
or cherries

2 tablespoons chia seeds

2 tablespoons monk fruit sweetener

4 teaspoons fresh lemon juice

Pinch of salt

2–3 mint leaves, chopped, optional

NOTES:

Use it up: Enjoy on toast, on oatmeal, in yogurt parfaits, over ice cream, and more!

Store leftovers: Refrigerate in an airtight container for up to a week.

No monk fruit sweetener? Use two chopped dates instead.

Reduce food waste: Use leftover mint in the Epic Rainbow Fruit Salad (page 211).

Makes 1 cup   ○ Cooking Time: 10 minutes, plus 30 minutes rest time

Unlike typical jams, this version uses chia seeds to create a gel-like consistency. Chia seeds are also full of fiber, which helps balance blood sugar and improves insulin sensitivity. Monk fruit adds sweetness while keeping the jam blood sugar-friendly.

1. Thaw the berries in a saucepan over medium heat. When softened, mash with a fork or spatula.

2. Stir in the chia seeds, monk fruit sweetener, lemon juice and salt. Remove from the heat and let sit at room temperature for 30 minutes for the chia seeds to gel, stirring once halfway through.

3. Transfer to a jar.

*Nutrition information is per serving

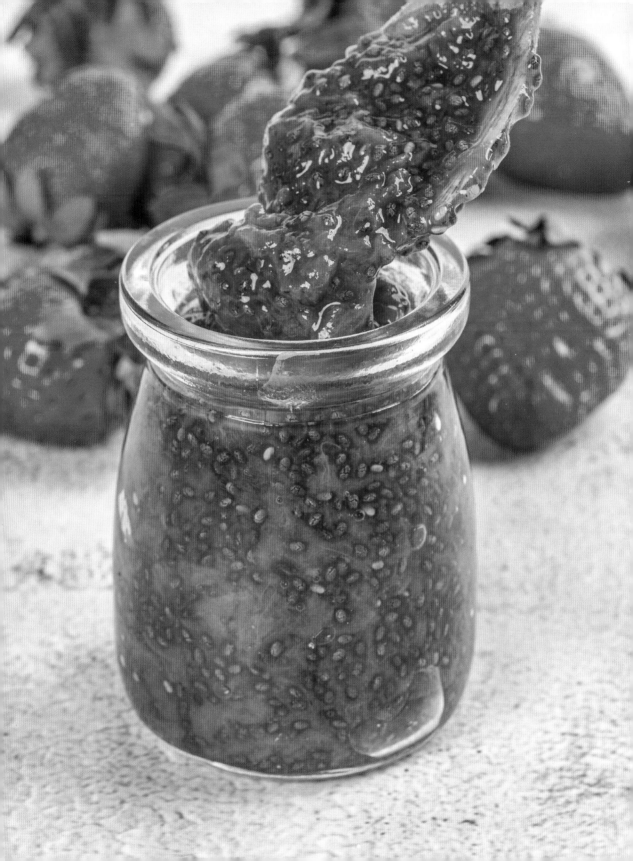

Eggless Mayo

Per 2 tablespoons: Calories: 32 | Fat: 2g | Carbs: 1g | Fiber: 0g | Protein: 2g

1 (12-ounce) carton silken tofu, extra firm

¼ cup aquafaba (liquid from a can of chickpeas)

2 teaspoons Dijon mustard

½ tablespoon fresh lemon juice

½ tablespoon apple cider vinegar

½ tablespoon olive oil

1 garlic clove

½ teaspoon salt

Makes 2 cups   🕐 Cooking Time: 5 minutes

Aquafaba is the thick liquid surrounding cooked chickpeas in a can. It has similar functional properties to eggs, making it a good substitute for eggs in many recipes. This recipe uses aquafaba and tofu to make a plant-based mayo that's low in calories and contains no saturated fat.

1. In a high-speed blender or food processor, blend all the ingredients until completely smooth.

NOTES:

Store leftovers: Refrigerate in an airtight container for up to five days.

Cashew Sour Cream

Per 2 tablespoons: Calories: 80 | Fat: 6g | Carbs: 5g | Fiber: 1g | Protein: 2g

1 cup raw cashews

2 tablespoons apple cider vinegar

1 tablespoon fresh lemon juice

¼ teaspoon salt

Makes 1-1½ cups   🕐 Cooking Time: 5 minutes

Cashews are a great base for sauces. Here, we blend cashews with water and seasoning to create a creamy, cheese-like sauce full of healthy fats. What's more, cashews may even help improve insulin resistance, making this alternative sour cream a better option for diabetes management.

NOTES:

Make it nut-free: Use sunflower or pumpkin seeds in place of the cashews. You may need to increase the amount of water to achieve the desired thickness.

Store leftovers: Refrigerate in an airtight container for up to five days.

1. Combine all the ingredients with ½ cup water in a high-speed blender and blend until smooth, stopping to scrape down the sides as necessary.

2. Serve immediately or chill for later use.

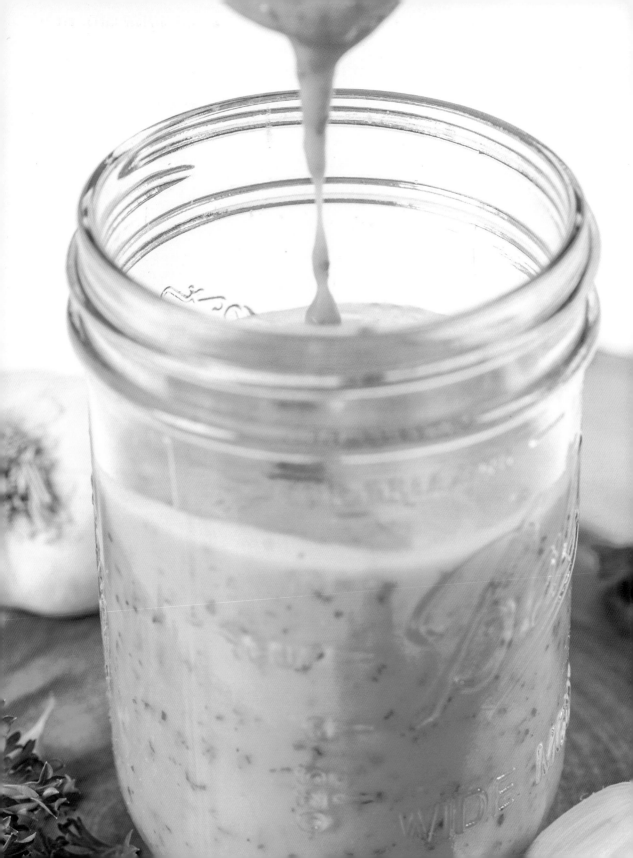

Green Goddess Drizzle

Per ¼ cup: Calories: 89 | Fat: 8g | Carbs: 6g | Fiber: 4g | Protein: 2g

1 cup chopped fresh parsley

1 ripe medium avocado

1 garlic clove

2 tablespoons chopped fresh basil

½ tablespoon fresh lemon juice

½ tablespoon apple cider vinegar

½ teaspoon salt

½ teaspoon onion powder

¼ teaspoon black pepper

Makes 1 cup   ○ Cooking Time: 10 minutes

This low-carb recipe uses avocado instead of oil to provide a creamy texture. It's perfect for topping any salad, bowl, or dinner.

1. In a high-speed blender or food processor, blend all the ingredients with ¼ cup water until smooth, scraping down the sides as needed.

NOTES:

Store leftovers: Store in an airtight container in the refrigerator for three to four days.

Creamy Balsamic Vinaigrette

Per 2 tablespoons: Calories: 103 | Fat: 8g | Carbs: 6g | Fiber: 1g | Protein: 3g

1 cup cashews

3 tablespoons balsamic vinegar

1 teaspoon dried oregano

½ teaspoon salt

½ teaspoon black pepper

NOTES:

Make it nut-free: Use sunflower seeds instead of cashews and an extra ½ cup water.

Store leftovers: Refrigerate in an airtight container for up to five days.

Makes 1 cup   ◷ Cooking Time: 5 minutes

Our take on the classic balsamic vinaigrette uses cashews to create a creamy, oil-free dressing beneficial for balancing your blood sugar.

1. In a high-speed blender or food processor, blend all the ingredients with ½ cup of water until smooth, scraping down the sides as needed.

*Nutrition information is per serving

Creamy Orange-Ginger Dressing

Per 2 tablespoons: Calories: 64 | Fat: 5g | Carbs: 4g | Fiber: 1g | Protein: 2g

¼ cup freshly squeezed orange juice (from 2 oranges)

¼ cup rice vinegar

3 tablespoons tahini

2 teaspoons miso

1 garlic clove

1 teaspoon minced ginger

½ teaspoon monk fruit sweetener or ½ Medjool date

Makes ⅔ cup   🕐 Cooking Time: 5 minutes

Miso is a thick paste made of fermented soybeans mixed with salt. Miso provides a salty, umami flavor to dishes and adds depth to dressings, and it may also help with reducing insulin resistance.

1. In a high-speed blender or food processor, blend all the ingredients until smooth.

NOTES:

Shop smart: Be sure to use freshly squeezed orange juice, as store-bought orange juice changes the taste of this recipe.

Make it soy-free: Omit the miso from the recipe.

Store leftovers: Refrigerate in an airtight container for up to five days.

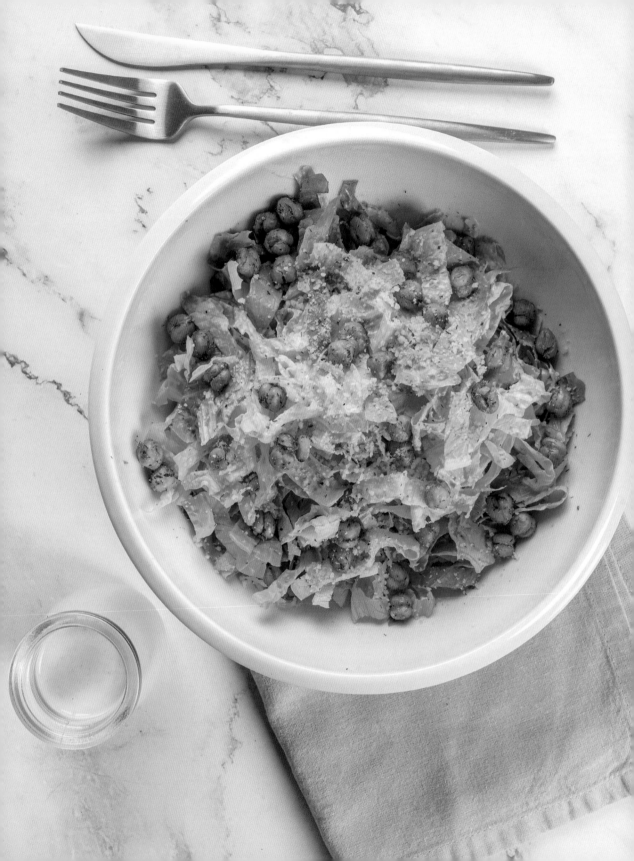

Tahini Caesar Dressing

Per 2 tablespoons: Calories: 93 | Fat: 8g | Carbs: 4g | Fiber: 1g | Protein: 3g

¼ cup tahini

2 tablespoons fresh lemon juice

1 garlic clove

1 teaspoon capers

2 teaspoons caper brine (from the jar of capers)

1 teaspoon Dijon mustard

1 teaspoon nutritional yeast

¼ teaspoon salt

Black pepper, to taste

Makes ½ cup   🕐 Cooking Time: 5 minutes

This blood sugar-friendly, plant-based Caesar keeps the tanginess of the classic dressing but without the dairy and saturated fat. The capers add a tangy, salty taste that mimics the flavor of the anchovies traditionally found in a Caesar salad.

1. In a blender, combine all the ingredients and blend until smooth.

2. Add 3 tablespoons or more of water to thin out the dressing to your preferred consistency.

NOTES:

Store leftovers: Refrigerate in an airtight container for up to five days. Add more water to thin out the dressing if it thickens in the fridge.

*Nutrition information is per serving

Appendix: Our Favorite Brands

If you're new to plant-based eating, choosing the right ingredients and decoding labels can feel overwhelming at first. Below you'll find a few of our favorite brands for categories that can be trickier to navigate. **Note:** this is not a comprehensive list, just a few of our favorite brands.

Whole-Grain Cereals

- Food for Life Ezekiel 4:9 cereal
- Uncle Sam cereal
- Grape-Nuts
- Engine 2 Plant-Strong cereal
- One Degree Organic Foods Sprouted Brown Rice Crisps
- Nature's Path cereal

Whole-Grain Crackers

- Mary's Gone Crackers (Original or Super Seed varieties)
- Triscuit Reduced Fat Whole Grain Wheat Crackers
- Wasa crackers
- Flackers
- Trader Joe's Crispbread
- FINN CRISP crackers
- Lundberg Brown Rice Cakes
- Lundberg Brown Rice Thin Stackers

Whole-Grain Bread

- Food For Life Ezekiel 4:9 Bread
- Alvarado St. Bakery
- Mighty Manna Bread
- Mestemacher
- Silver Hills Sprouted Power

Tortillas

- Food for Life Sprouted Corn Tortillas
- Food for Life Ezekiel 4:9 Sprouted Grain Tortillas
- Engine 2 Plant-Strong Sprouted Ancient Grains

Veggie Burgers

Aim for varieties with at least 6 grams of protein per patty

- Engine 2 Plant-Strong Burgers
- Dr. Praeger's Burgers
- Amy's Veggie Burgers
- Hilary's Burgers

Monk Fruit Sweetener

- Splenda Naturals Monk Fruit
- Lakanto Monk Fruit Sweetener

No-Sugar-Added Chocolate

- LILY'S chocolate
- Lakanto chocolate
- Hu No Added Sugar chocolate
- Serwe Dark Chocolate
- Taza Dark Chocolate

Salt Alternatives

- Mrs. Dash
- Kingsford Original No Salt All-Purpose Seasoning
- Chef Paul Prudhomme's Magic Seasoning Blends
- Magic Salt-Free Seasoning
- Spike Gourmet Natural Seasoning
- Loisa Salt-Free Adobo
- Flavor Mate No Salt Seasoning
- Everything But the Salt Seasoning by Flavor God

Non-Dairy Yogurt

- Kite Hill Plain Unsweetened Almond Milk Yogurt
- Kite Hill Plain Unsweetened Greek Style Yogurt
- Kite Hill Vanilla Unsweetened Greek Style Yogurt
- So Delicious Unsweetened Plain Coconut Milk Yogurt
- Silk Unsweetened Vanilla Almond Milk Yogurt
- DAH! Plain Almond Yogurt
- LAVA Pili Nut Yogurt (any flavor)

Non-Dairy Creamers

- Califia Farms Unsweetened Better Half half-and-half substitute
- Califia Farms Unsweetened Almondmilk Creamer
- Califia Farms Unsweetened Oat Creamer
- Nutpods unsweetened creamers
- Elmhurst Unsweetened Oat Creamer

Protein Powders

- Garden of Life Raw Organic Protein
- Sunwarrior Protein Warrior Blend
- Sprout Living Simple Sunflower Seed Protein
- Hemp Yeah! Unsweetened
- Nutiva Hemp Protein
- Naked PB
- Truvani
- Orgain Organic Pea Protein

Protein / Snack Bars

- No Cow Protein Bars
- IQBARs
- Garden of Life Organic Fit Bars
- Health Warrior Chia Bars
- KIND Minis
- Raw Rev Bars

References

FRONT MATTER

Introduction

"...537 million people globally, and is expected to rise to 643 million by 2030." (Page 5):
International Diabetes Federation. (2021). IDF Diabetes Atlas 10th Edition. Retrieved from https://diabetesatlas.org/idfawp/resource-files/2021/07/IDF_Atlas_10th_Edition_2021.pdf

"...eighth leading cause of death and number one cause of kidney failure, lower-limb amputations, and adult blindness." (Page 5):
Centers for Disease Control and Prevention. (2021). Diabetes Basics. Retrieved from https://www.cdc.gov/diabetes/basics/diabetes.html

"...the Journal of the Association of American Medical Colleges..." (Page 7):
Adams, K. M., Lindell, K. C., Kohlmeier, M., Zeisel, S. H. (2010). Nutrition Education in US Medical Schools: Latest Update of a National Survey. Academic Medicine, 85(9), 1537-1542. https://doi.org/10.1097/ACM.0b013e3181eab71b

"...lasts a mere 20 minutes." (Page 7):
Irving G, Neves AL, Dambha-Miller H, et alInternational variations in primary care physician consultation time: a systematic review of 67 countriesBMJ Open 2017;7:e017902. doi: 10.1136/bmjopen-2017-017902

CHAPTER 1

Diagnosis

"...diagnosed through the several tests..." (Page 14):

Nuha A. ElSayed, Grazia Aleppo, Vanita R. Aroda, Raveendhara R. Bannuru, Florence M. Brown, Dennis Bruemmer, Billy S. Collins, Marisa E. Hilliard, Diana Isaacs, Eric L. Johnson, Scott Kahan, Kamlesh Khunti, Jose Leon, Sarah K. Lyons, Mary Lou Perry, Priya Prahalad, Richard E. Pratley, Jane Jeffrie Seley, Robert C. Stanton, Robert A. Gabbay; on behalf of the American Diabetes Association, 2. Classification and Diagnosis of Diabetes: Standards of Care in Diabetes—2023. Diabetes Care 1 January 2023; 46 (Supplement_1): S19–S40. https://doi.org/10.2337/dc23-S002

How Insulin Resistance Leads to Type 2 Diabetes

"...significantly improves insulin sensitivity..." (Page 18):

Risérus, U., Willett, W. C., & Hu, F. B. (2009). Dietary fats and prevention of type 2 diabetes. Progress in lipid research, 48(1), 44–51. https://doi.org/10.1016/j.plipres.2008.10.002

Imamura, F., Micha, R., Wu, J. H., de Oliveira Otto, M. C., Otite, F. O., Abioye, A. I., & Mozaffarian, D. (2016). Effects of Saturated Fat, Polyunsaturated Fat, Monounsaturated Fat, and Carbohydrate on Glucose-Insulin Homeostasis: A Systematic Review and Meta-analysis of Randomised Controlled Feeding Trials. PLoS medicine, 13(7), e1002087. https://doi.org/10.1371/journal.pmed.1002087

"...96 million Americans (more than 1 in 3) have prediabetes..." (Page 19)
Centers for Disease Control and Prevention. (2021). Prediabetes. Retrieved from https://www.cdc.gov/diabetes/basics/prediabetes.html

"... affects 33 to 35 million Americans." (Page 19):
Centers for Disease Control and Prevention. (2021). Type 2 Diabetes. Retrieved from https://www.cdc.gov/diabetes/basics/type2.html

"...2002 Diabetes Prevention Program trial..." (Page 19):
Knowler, W. C., Barrett-Connor, E., Fowler, S. E., Hamman, R. F., Lachin, J. M., Walker, E. A., Nathan, D. M., & Diabetes Prevention Program Research Group (2002). Reduction in the incidence of type 2 diabetes with lifestyle intervention or metformin. The New England journal of medicine, 346(6), 393–403. https://doi.org/10.1056/NEJMoa012512

What Increases Your Risk of Prediabetes and Type 2 Diabetes?

"..strongest risk factors for type 2 diabetes..." (Page 20):
Nuha A. ElSayed, Grazia Aleppo, Vanita R. Aroda, Raveendhara R. Bannuru, Florence M. Brown, Dennis Bruemmer, Billy S. Collins, Marisa E. Hilliard, Diana Isaacs, Eric L. Johnson, Scott Kahan, Kamlesh Khunti, Jose Leon, Sarah K. Lyons, Mary Lou Perry, Priya Prahalad, Richard E. Pratley, Jane Jeffrie Seley, Robert C. Stanton, Robert A. Gabbay; on behalf of the American Diabetes Association, 2. Classification and Diagnosis of Diabetes: Standards of Care in Diabetes—2023. Diabetes Care 1 January 2023; 46 (Supplement_1): S19–S40. https://doi.org/10.2337/dc23-S002

"...common risk factors..." (Page 20):
Centers for Disease Control and Prevention. (2021). Diabetes Risk Factors. Retrieved from https://www.cdc.gov/diabetes/basics/risk-factors.html

"..genetics of type 2 diabetes are still poorly understood." (Page 20):

Nuha A. ElSayed, Grazia Aleppo, Vanita R. Aroda, Raveendhara R. Bannuru, Florence M. Brown, Dennis Bruemmer, Billy S. Collins, Marisa E. Hilliard, Diana Isaacs, Eric L. Johnson, Scott Kahan, Kamlesh Khunti, Jose Leon, Sarah K. Lyons, Mary Lou Perry, Priya Prahalad, Richard E. Pratley, Jane Jeffrie Seley, Robert C. Stanton, Robert A. Gabbay; on behalf of the American Diabetes Association, 2. Classification and Diagnosis of Diabetes: Standards of Care in Diabetes—2023. Diabetes Care 1 January 2023; 46 (Supplement_1): S19–S40. https://doi.org/10.2337/dc23-S002

Long-Term Complications of Type 2 Diabetes

"...twice as likely to have a heart attack or stroke... (Page 21):
Centers for Disease Control and Prevention. (2021). Diabetes and Heart Disease. Retrieved from https://www.cdc.gov/diabetes/library/features/diabetes-and-heart.html

"...more than 65% of people with type 2 diabetes..." (Page 21):
Laakso M. (2010). Cardiovascular disease in type 2 diabetes from population to man to mechanisms: the Kelly West Award Lecture 2008. Diabetes care, 33(2), 442–449. https://doi.org/10.2337/dc09-0749

"...leading cause of kidney disease..." (Page 21):
National Institute of Diabetes and Digestive and Kidney Diseases. (2021). Diabetic Kidney Disease. Retrieved from https://www.niddk.nih.gov/health-information/diabetes/overview/preventing-problems/diabetic-kidney-disease

"...affects nearly half of all diabetes sufferers..." (Page 21):
National Institute of Diabetes and Digestive and Kidney Diseases. (2021). Peripheral Neuropathy. Retrieved from https://www.niddk.nih.gov/health-information/diabetes/overview/preventing-problems/nerve-damage-diabetic-neuropathies/peripheral-neuropathy

"...more than 30% of people..." (Page 21):
National Institute of Diabetes and Digestive and Kidney Diseases. (2021). What is Diabetic Neuropathy? Retrieved from https://www.niddk.nih.gov/health-information/diabetes/overview/preventing-problems/nerve-damage-diabetic-neuropathies/what-is-diabetic-neuropathy

"...lead to amputations." (Page 21):
National Institute of Diabetes and Digestive and Kidney Diseases. (2021). Foot Problems. Retrieved from https://www.niddk.nih.gov/health-information/diabetes/overview/preventing-problems/foot-problems

"...leading causes of amputations..." (Page 21):
Molina CS, Faulk JB. Lower Extremity Amputation. [Updated 2022 Aug 22]. In: StatPearls [Internet]. Treasure Island (FL):

StatPearls Publishing; 2023 Jan-. Available from: https://www.ncbi.nlm.nih.gov/books/NBK546594/

"...leading to blurred vision." (Page 21):
Centers for Disease Control and Prevention. (2021). Diabetes and Vision Loss. Retrieved from https://www.cdc.gov/diabetes/managing/diabetes-vision-loss.html

Can Type 2 Diabetes Be Reversed or Put Into Remission

"The Counterpoint, Counterbalance, and DiRECT trials..." (Page 22):
Singla, R., Gupta, G., Dutta, D., Raizada, N., & Aggarwal, S. (2022). Diabetes reversal: Update on current knowledge and proposal of prediction score parameters for diabetes remission. Diabetes & metabolic syndrome, 16(4), 102452. https://doi.org/10.1016/j.dsx.2022.102452

"The American Diabetes Association (ADA) says..." (Page 22):
American Diabetes Association Professional Practice Committee; 5. Facilitating Behavior Change and Well-being to Improve Health Outcomes: Standards of Medical Care in Diabetes—2022. Diabetes Care 1 January 2022; 45 (Supplement_1): S60–S82. https://doi.org/10.2337/dc22-S005

"Based on the ample research available..." (Page 22):
Kirkpatrick, C. F., Bolick, J. P., Kris-Etherton, P. M., Sikand, G., Aspry, K. E., Soffer, D. E., Willard, K. E., & Maki, K. C. (2019). Review of current evidence and clinical recommendations on the effects of low-carbohydrate and very-low-carbohydrate (including ketogenic) diets for the management of body weight and other cardiometabolic risk factors: A scientific statement from the National Lipid Association Nutrition and Lifestyle Task Force. Journal of clinical lipidology, 13(5), 689–711.e1. https://doi.org/10.1016/j.jacl.2019.08.003

"...more difficult to stick to in the long-term..." (Page 22):
American Diabetes Association Professional Practice Committee; 5. Facilitating Behavior Change and Well-being to Improve Health Outcomes: Standards of Medical Care in Diabetes—2022. Diabetes Care 1 January 2022; 45 (Supplement_1): S60–S82. https://doi.org/10.2337/dc22-S005

CHAPTER 2

Nutrient Density vs Calorie Density

"...can lead to excess weight—a contributor of insulin resistance. " (Page 26):
Nuha A. ElSayed, Grazia Aleppo, Vanita R. Aroda, Raveendhara R. Bannuru, Florence M. Brown, Dennis Bruemmer, Billy S. Collins, Marisa E. Hilliard, Diana Isaacs,

Eric L. Johnson, Scott Kahan, Kamlesh Khunti, Jose Leon, Sarah K. Lyons, Mary Lou Perry, Priya Prahalad, Richard E. Pratley, Jane Jeffrie Seley, Robert C. Stanton, Robert A. Gabbay; on behalf of the American Diabetes Association, 2. Classification and Diagnosis of Diabetes: Standards of Care in Diabetes—2023. Diabetes Care 1 January 2023; 46 (Supplement_1): S19–S40. https://doi.org/10.2337/dc23-S002

"Dan Buettner teamed up with National Geographic..." (Page 27):
Buettner, Dan. He Blue Zones Solution: Eating and Living Like the World's Healthiest People. National Geographic Society, 2015.

"...reduce the risk to type 2 diabetes, treat type 2 diabetes, and reduce key diabetes-related complications." (Page 27):
Rinaldi S, Campbell EE, Fournier J, O'Connor C, Madill J. A comprehensive review of the literature supporting recommendations from the Canadian Diabetes Association for the use of a plant-based diet for management of type 2 diabetes. Can J Diabetes 2016;40:471–477

de Carvalho GB, Dias-Vasconcelos NL, Santos RKF, Brandao-Lima PN, da Silva DG, Pires LV. Effect of different dietary patterns on glycemic control in individuals with type 2 diabetes mellitus: a systematic review. Crit Rev Food Sci Nutr 2020;60:1999–2010

Papamichou D, Panagiotakos DB, Itsiopoulos C. Dietary patterns and management of type 2 diabetes: a systematic review of randomised clinical trials. Nutr Metab Cardiovasc Dis 2019;29: 531–543

Pawlak R. Vegetarian diets in the prevention and management of diabetes and its complications. Diabetes Spectr 2017;30:82–88

"The American Diabetes Association's 2023 Standards of Care..." (Page 27):
American Diabetes Association Professional Practice Committee; 5. Facilitating Behavior Change and Well-being to Improve Health Outcomes: Standards of Medical Care in Diabetes—2022. Diabetes Care 1 January 2022; 45 (Supplement_1): S60–S82. https://doi.org/10.2337/dc22-S005

"...2021 Dietary Guidance to Improve Cardiovascular Health..." (Page 27):
Lichtenstein, A. H., Appel, L. J., Vadiveloo, M., Hu, F. B., Kris-Etherton, P. M., Rebholz, C. M., Sacks, F. M., Thorndike, A. N., Van Horn, L., & Wylie-Rosett, J. (2021). 2021 Dietary Guidance to Improve Cardiovascular Health: A Scientific Statement From the American Heart Association. Circulation, 144(23), e472–e487. https://doi.org/10.1161/CIR.0000000000001031

"..American Association of Clinical Endocrinology..." (Page 27):
American Association of Clinical Endocrinologists. (2021). AACE 2019 Diabetes Algorithm. Retrieved from https://pro.aace.com/pdfs/diabetes/AACE_2019_Diabetes_Algorithm_03.2021.pdf

"...American College of Lifestyle Medicine...(Page 27):
Rosenfeld RM, Kelly JH, Agarwal M, et al. Dietary Interventions to Treat Type 2 Diabetes in Adults with a Goal of Remission: An Expert Consensus Statement from the American College of Lifestyle Medicine. American Journal of Lifestyle Medicine. 2022;16(3):342-362. doi:10.1177/15598276221087624

The Elements of a Plant-Based Diet for Type 2 Diabetes

"...improve glycemic control and insulin sensitivity." (Page 28):
Fu, L., Zhang, G., Qian, S., Zhang, Q., & Tan, M. (2022). Associations between dietary fiber intake and cardiovascular risk factors: An umbrella review of meta-analyses of randomized controlled trials. Frontiers in nutrition, 9, 972399. https://doi.org/10.3389/fnut.2022.972399

Kim, Y., Keogh, J. B., & Clifton, P. M. (2016). Polyphenols and Glycemic Control. Nutrients, 8(1), 17. https://doi.org/10.3390/nu8010017

"...improves HbA1c, fasting blood sugar, fasting insulin, and insulin resistance."
Fu, L., Zhang, G., Qian, S., Zhang, Q., & Tan, M. (2022). Associations between dietary fiber intake and cardiovascular risk factors: An umbrella review of meta-analyses of randomized controlled trials. Frontiers in nutrition, 9, 972399. https://doi.org/10.3389/fnut.2022.972399

"...promotes satiety and has been linked with weight loss..." (Page 28):
Lattimer, J. M., & Haub, M. D. (2010). Effects of dietary fiber and its components on metabolic health. Nutrients, 2(12), 1266–1289. https://doi.org/10.3390/nu2121266

"...improve glucose response, insulin signaling, insulin sensitivity, and pancreatic dysfunction." (Page 28)
Puddu, A., Sanguineti, R., Montecucco, F., & Viviani, G. L. (2014). Evidence for the gut microbiota short-chain fatty acids as key pathophysiological molecules improving diabetes. Mediators of inflammation, 2014, 162021. https://doi.org/10.1155/2014/162021

Mandaliya, D. K., & Seshadri, S. (2019). Short Chain Fatty Acids, pancreatic dysfunction and type 2 diabetes. Pancreatology : official journal of the International Association of Pancreatology (IAP) ... [et al.], 19(2), 280–284. https://doi.org/10.1016/j.pan.2019.01.021

Tilg, H., & Moschen, A. R. (2014). Microbiota and diabetes: an evolving relationship. Gut, 63(9), 1513–1521. https://doi.org/10.1136/gutjnl-2014-306928

Baothman, O. A., Zamzami, M. A., Taher, I., Abubaker, J., & Abu-Farha, M. (2016). The role of Gut Microbiota in the development of obesity and Diabetes. Lipids in health and disease, 15, 108. https://doi.org/10.1186/s12944-016-0278-4

"...associated with reducing markers of inflammation." (Page 28)
Fu, L., Zhang, G., Qian, S., Zhang, Q., & Tan, M. (2022). Associations between dietary fiber intake and cardiovascular risk factors: An umbrella review of meta-analyses of randomized controlled trials. Frontiers in nutrition, 9, 972399. https://doi.org/10.3389/fnut.2022.972399

"...only 7% of Americans..." (Page 28):
Miketinas, D. C., Tucker, W. J., Douglas, C. C., & Patterson, M. A. (2023). Usual Dietary Fiber Intake According to Diabetes Status in US Adults: NHANES 2013-2018. The British journal of nutrition, 1–26. Advance online publication. https://doi.org/10.1017/S0007114523000089

"...stimulate insulin secretion and improve the uptake of glucose into cells." (Page 28)
Kim, Y., Keogh, J. B., & Clifton, P. M. (2016). Polyphenols and Glycemic Control. Nutrients, 8(1), 17. https://doi.org/10.3390/nu8010017

"...have not been shown to prevent disease." (Page 28)
National Center for Complementary and Integrative Health. (2021). Antioxidants in Depth. Retrieved from https://www.nccih.nih.gov/health/antioxidants-in-depth

"...linked to insulin resistance and an increased risk of type 2 diabetes." (Page 29)
Xiao, C., Giacca, A., Carpentier, A., & Lewis, G. F. (2006). Differential effects of monounsaturated, polyunsaturated and saturated fat ingestion on glucose-stimulated insulin secretion, sensitivity and clearance in overweight and obese, non-diabetic humans. Diabetologia, 49(6), 1371–1379. https://doi.org/10.1007/s00125-006-0211-x

Wang, L., Folsom, A. R., Zheng, Z. J., Pankow, J. S., Eckfeldt, J. H., & ARIC Study Investigators (2003). Plasma fatty acid composition and incidence of diabetes in middle-aged adults: the Atherosclerosis Risk in Communities (ARIC) Study. The American journal of clinical nutrition, 78(1), 91–98. https://doi.org/10.1093/ajcn/78.1.91

von Frankenberg, A. D., Marina, A., Song, X., Callahan, H. S., Kratz, M., & Utzschneider, K. M. (2017). A high-fat, high-saturated fat diet decreases insulin sensitivity without changing intra-abdominal fat in weight-stable overweight and obese adults. European journal of nutrition, 56(1), 431–443. https://doi.org/10.1007/s00394-015-1108-6

Luukkonen, P. K., Sädevirta, S., Zhou, Y., Kayser, B., Ali, A., Ahonen, L., Lallukka, S., Pelloux, V., Gaggini, M., Jian, C., Hakkarainen, A., Lundbom, N., Gylling, H., Salonen, A., Orešič, M., Hyötyläinen, T., Orho-Melander, M., Rissanen, A., Gastaldelli, A., Clément, K., ... Yki-Järvinen, H. (2018). Saturated Fat Is More Metabolically Harmful for the Human Liver Than Unsaturated Fat or Simple Sugars. Diabetes care, 41(8), 1732–1739. https://doi.org/10.2337/dc18-0071

Riccardi, G., Giacco, R., & Rivellese, A. A. (2004). Dietary fat, insulin sensitivity and the metabolic syndrome. Clinical nutrition (Edinburgh, Scotland), 23(4), 447–456. https://doi.org/10.1016/j.clnu.2004.02.006

"Lipotoxicity impairs insulin signaling..." (Page 29)
Ertunc, M. E., & Hotamisligil, G. S. (2016). Lipid signaling and lipotoxicity in metaflammation: indications for metabolic disease pathogenesis and treatment. Journal of lipid research, 57(12), 2099–2114. https://doi.org/10.1194/jlr.R066514

Nolan, C. J., & Larter, C. Z. (2009). Lipotoxicity: why do saturated fatty acids cause and monounsaturates protect against it?. Journal of gastroenterology and hepatology, 24(5), 703–706. https://doi.org/10.1111/j.1440-1746.2009.05823.x

Estadella, D., da Penha Oller do Nascimento, C. M., Oyama, L. M., Ribeiro, E. B., Dâmaso, A. R., & de Piano, A. (2013). Lipotoxicity: effects of dietary saturated and transfatty acids. Mediators of inflammation, 2013, 137579. https://doi.org/10.1155/2013/137579

"...unsaturated fat can improve glycemic control..." (Page 29):
Imamura, F., Micha, R., Wu, J. H., de Oliveira Otto, M. C., Otite, F. O., Abioye, A. I., & Mozaffarian, D. (2016). Effects of Saturated Fat, Polyunsaturated Fat, Monounsaturated Fat, and Carbohydrate on Glucose-Insulin Homeostasis: A Systematic Review and Meta-analysis of Randomised Controlled Feeding Trials. PLoS medicine, 13(7), e1002087. https://doi.org/10.1371/journal.pmed.1002087

Vessby, B., Uusitupa, M., Hermansen, K., Riccardi, G., Rivellese, A. A., Tapsell, L. C., Nälsén, C., Berglund, L., Louheranta, A., Rasmussen, B. M., Calvert, G. D., Maffetone, A., Pedersen, E., Gustafsson, I. B., Storlien, L. H., & KANWU Study (2001). Substituting dietary saturated for monounsaturated fat impairs insulin sensitivity in healthy men and women: The KANWU Study. Diabetologia, 44(3), 312–319. https://doi.org/10.1007/s001250051620

"...promote weight and fat loss..." (Page 29):
Tonstad S, Butler T, Yan R, et al. Type of vegetarian diet, body weight, and prevalence of type 2 diabetes. Diabetes Care. 2009;32:791–796.

Spencer EA, Appleby PN, Davey GK, et al. Diet and body mass index in 38000 EPIC-Oxford meat-eaters, fish-eaters, vegetarians and vegans. Int J Obes Relat Metab Disord. 2003;27:728–734.

Turner-McGrievy GM, Davidson CR, Wingard EE, et al. Comparative effectiveness of plant-based diets for weight loss: a randomized controlled trial of five different diets. Nutrition. 2015;31:350–358.

Barnard ND, Levin SM, Yokoyama Y. A systematic review and meta-analysis of changes in body weight in clinical trials of vegetarian diets. J Acad Nutr Diet. 2015;115:954–969.

Huang RY, Huang CC, Hu FB, et al. Vegetarian diets and weight reduction: a meta-analysis of randomized controlled trials. J Gen Intern Med. 2016;31:109–116.

"...implicated in weight gain and insulin resistance." (Page 29):

Vang A, Singh PN, Lee JW, et al. Meats, processed meats, obesity, weight gain and occurrence of diabetes among adults: findings from Adventist Health Studies. Ann Nutr Metab. 2008;52:96–104.

Vergnaud AC. Meat consumption and prospective weight change in participants of the EPIC-PANACEA study. Am J Clin Nutr. 2010;92:398–407.

Vergnaud AC. Macronutrient composition of the diet and prospective weight change in participants of the EPIC-PANACEA study. PLoS One. 2013;8:e57300.

Wang Y, Beydoun MA. Meat consumption is associated with obesity and central obesity among US adults. Int J Obes (Lond) 2009;33:621–628.

Rosell M. Weight gain over 5 years in 21,966 meat-eating, fish-eating, vegetarian, and vegan men and women in EPIC-Oxford. Int J Obes. 2006;30:1389–1396.

Halkjaer J, Olsen A, Overvad K, et al. Intake of total, animal and plant protein and subsequent changes in weight or waist circumference in European men and women: the diogenes project. Int J Obes (Lond) 2011;35:1104–1113.

You W, Henneberg M. Meat consumption providing a surplus energy in modern diet contributes to obesity prevalence: an ecological analysis. BMC Nutrition. 2016;2:22.

AlEssa HB, Bhupathiraju SN, Malik VS, et al. Carbohydrate quality and quantity and risk of type 2 diabetes in US women. Am J Clin Nutr. 2015;102:1543–1553.

Malik VS, Hu FB. Fructose and cardiometabolic health: what the evidence from sugar-sweetened beverages tells us. J Am Coll Cardiol. 2015;66:1615–1624.

Bhupathiraju SN, Tobias DK, Malik VS, et al. Glycemic index, glycemic load, and risk of type 2 diabetes: results from 3 large US cohorts and an updated meta-analysis. Am J Clin Nutr. 2014;100:218–232

CHAPTER 3

Carb-to-Fiber Ratio

"...the Harvard School of Public Health..." (Page 40):

Mozaffarian, R., Lee, R., Kennedy, M., Ludwig, D., Mozaffarian, D., & Gortmaker, S. (2013). Identifying whole grain foods: A comparison of different approaches for selecting more healthful whole grain products. Public Health Nutrition, 16(12), 2255-2264. doi:10.1017/S1368980012005447

Tips for Success

"... improvements in eating control, body weight, HbA1c levels, and blood pressure." (Page 42):

Dasgupta, K., Hajna, S., Joseph, L., Da Costa, D., Christopoulos, S., & Gougeon, R. (2012). Effects of meal preparation training on body weight, glycemia, and blood pressure: results of a phase 2 trial in type 2 diabetes. The international journal of behavioral nutrition and physical activity, 9, 125. https://doi.org/10.1186/1479-5868-9-125

CHAPTER 4

What Can I Drink During the Meal Plan?

"...drink 9 to 13 cups..." (Page 51):
Harvard T.H. Chan School of Public Health. (2021). Water. Retrieved from https://www.hsph.harvard.edu/nutritionsource/water/

"...reduce your risk of type 2 diabetes." (Page 52):
Carlström, M., & Larsson, S. C. (2018). Coffee consumption and reduced risk of developing type 2 diabetes: a systematic review with meta-analysis. Nutrition reviews, 76(6), 395–417. https://doi.org/10.1093/nutrit/nuy014

"...American Heart Association (AHA)..." (Page 53):
American Heart Association. (2021). Added Sugars. Retrieved from https://www.heart.org/en/healthy-living/healthy-eating/eat-smart/sugar/added-sugars

Is Soy Safe To Eat?

"....decreased risk of prostate, GI, and breast cancer..." (Page 57):
Applegate, C. C., Rowles, J. L., Ranard, K. M., Jeon, S., & Erdman, J. W. (2018). Soy Consumption and the Risk of Prostate Cancer: An Updated Systematic Review and Meta-Analysis. Nutrients, 10(1), 40. https://doi.org/10.3390/nu10010040

Lu, D., Pan, C., Ye, C., Duan, H., Xu, F., Yin, L., Tian, W., & Zhang, S. (2017). Meta-analysis of Soy Consumption and Gastrointestinal Cancer Risk. Scientific reports, 7(1), 4048. https://doi.org/10.1038/s41598-017-03692-y

Tse, G., & Eslick, G. D. (2016). Soy and isoflavone consumption and risk of gastrointestinal cancer: a systematic review and meta-analysis. European journal of nutrition, 55(1), 63–73. https://doi.org/10.1007/s00394-014-0824-7

Boutas, I., Kontogeorgi, A., Dimitrakakis, C., & Kalantaridou, S. N. (2022). Soy Isoflavones and Breast Cancer Risk: A Meta-analysis. In vivo (Athens, Greece), 36(2), 556–562. https://doi.org/10.21873/invivo.12737

"...decreased risk of type 2 diabetes..." (Page 57):
Li, W., Ruan, W., Peng, Y., & Wang, D. (2018). Soy and the risk of type 2 diabetes mellitus: A systematic review and meta-analysis of observational studies. Diabetes research and clinical practice, 137, 190–199. https://doi.org/10.1016/j.diabres.2018.01.010

"...prevent osteoporosis, or the weakening of bones." (Page 57)
Castelo-Branco, C., & Cancelo Hidalgo, M. J. (2011). Isoflavones: effects on bone health. Climacteric : the journal of the International Menopause Society, 14(2), 204–211. https://doi.org/10.3109/13697137.2010.529198

"...improve your cholesterol and body weight" (Page 57):
Taku, K., Umegaki, K., Sato, Y., Taki, Y., Endoh, K., & Watanabe, S. (2007). Soy isoflavones lower serum total and LDL cholesterol in humans: a meta-analysis of 11 randomized controlled trials. The American journal of clinical nutrition, 85(4), 1148–1156. https://doi.org/10.1093/ajcn/85.4.1148

Zhang, Y. B., Chen, W. H., Guo, J. J., Fu, Z. H., Yi, C., Zhang, M., & Na, X. L. (2013). Soy isoflavone supplementation could reduce body weight and improve glucose metabolism in non-Asian postmenopausal women—a meta-analysis. Nutrition (Burbank, Los Angeles County, Calif.), 29(1), 8–14. https://doi.org/10.1016/j.nut.2012.03.019

Do I Need To Be Concerned With Salt/Sodium?

"...for heart disease and stroke." (Page 58)
Centers for Disease Control and Prevention. (2021). Sodium and Salt. Retrieved from https://www.cdc.gov/heartdisease/sodium.htm

"..top 10 sources of sodium..." (Page 58):
Centers for Disease Control and Prevention. (2021). Sources of Sodium. Retrieved from https://www.cdc.gov/salt/food.htm

"...American Heart Association recommends..." (Page 58):
American Heart Association. (2016). Why Should I Limit Sodium? Retrieved from https://www.heart.org/-/media/files/health-topics/answers-by-heart/why-should-i-limit-sodium.pdf

How Will the Meal Plan Affect My Budget

"reduce food costs by over 30%." (Page 61)
Springmann, M., Clark, M. A., Rayner, M., Scarborough, P., & Webb, P. (2021). The global and regional costs of healthy and sustainable dietary patterns: a modelling study. The Lancet. Planetary health, 5(11), e797–e807. https://doi.org/10.1016/S2542-5196(21)00251-5

CHAPTER 6

"The Adventist Health Study 2..." (Page 95):
Tonstad, S., Butler, T., Yan, R., & Fraser, G. E. (2009). Type of vegetarian diet, body weight, and prevalence of type 2 diabetes. Diabetes care, 32(5), 791–796. https://doi.org/10.2337/dc08-1886

"improve glycemic control and HbA1c..." (Page 97)
Hyun, M. K., Lee, J. W., Ko, S. H., & Hwang, J. S. (2022). Improving Glycemic Control in Type 2 Diabetes Using Mobile Applications and e-Coaching: A Mixed Treatment Comparison Network Meta-Analysis. Journal of diabetes science and technology, 16(5), 1239–1252. https://doi.org/10.1177/19322968211010153

"...virtual coaching aids..." (Page 97):
Shen, Y., Wang, F., Zhang, X., Zhu, X., Sun, Q., Fisher, E., & Sun, X. (2018). Effectiveness of Internet-Based Interventions on Glycemic Control in Patients With Type 2 Diabetes: Meta-Analysis of Randomized Controlled Trials. Journal of medical Internet research, 20(5), e172. https://doi.org/10.2196/jmir.9133

"Group programs create...'" (Page 97):
Steinsbekk, A., Rygg, L. Ø., Lisulo, M., Rise, M. B., & Fretheim, A. (2012). Group based diabetes self-management education compared to routine treatment for people with type 2 diabetes mellitus. A systematic review with meta-analysis. BMC health services research, 12, 213. https://doi.org/10.1186/1472-6963-12-213

"...multidisciplinary team..." (Page 98):
Centers for Disease Control and Prevention. (2021). Multidisciplinary Diabetes Self-Management Education and Support (DSMES) Team. Retrieved from https://www.cdc.gov/diabetes/dsmes-toolkit/staffing-delivery/multidisciplinary-dsmes-team.html

"Physical activity can lead to..." (Page 99):
Schuch, F. B., Vancampfort, D., Firth, J., Rosenbaum, S., Ward, P. B., Silva, E. S., Hallgren, M., Ponce De Leon, A., Dunn, A. L., Deslandes, A. C., Fleck, M. P., Carvalho, A. F., & Stubbs, B. (2018). Physical Activity and Incident Depression: A Meta-Analysis of Prospective Cohort Studies. The American journal of psychiatry, 175(7), 631–648. https://doi.org/10.1176/appi.ajp.2018.17111194

de Kam, D., Smulders, E., Weerdesteyn, V., & Smits-Engelsman, B. C. (2009). Exercise interventions to reduce fall-related fractures and their risk factors in individuals with low bone density: a systematic review of randomized controlled trials. Osteoporosis international : a journal established as result of cooperation between the European Foundation for Osteoporosis and the National Osteoporosis Foundation of the USA, 20(12), 2111–2125. https://doi.org/10.1007/s00198-009-0938-6

Batrakoulis, A., Jamurtas, A. Z., Metsios, G. S., Perivoliotis, K., Liguori, G., Feito, Y., Riebe, D., Thompson, W. R., Angelopoulos, T. J., Krustrup, P., Mohr, M., Draganidis, D., Poulios, A., & Fatouros, I. G. (2022). Comparative Efficacy of 5 Exercise Types on Cardiometabolic Health in Overweight and Obese Adults: A Systematic Review and Network Meta-Analysis of 81 Randomized Controlled Trials. Circulation. Cardiovascular quality and outcomes, 15(6), e008243. https://doi.org/10.1161/CIRCOUTCOMES.121.008243

"...impact on your blood sugar." (Page 99):
Pahra, D., Sharma, N., Ghai, S., Hajela, A., Bhansali, S., & Bhansali, A. (2017). Impact of post-meal and one-time daily exercise in patient with type 2 diabetes mellitus: a randomized crossover study. Diabetology & metabolic syndrome, 9, 64. https://doi.org/10.1186/s13098-017-0263-8

"...higher incidence of insulin resistance and type 2 diabetes." (Page 99):
Perry, B. D., Caldow, M. K., Brennan-Speranza, T. C., Sbaraglia, M., Jerums, G., Garnham, A., Wong, C., Levinger, P., Asrar Ul Haq, M., Hare, D. L., Price, S. R., & Levinger, I. (2016). Muscle atrophy in patients with Type 2 Diabetes Mellitus: roles of inflammatory pathways, physical activity and exercise. Exercise immunology review, 22, 94–109.

"...blood glucose elevated and may lead to..." (Page 100):
Yaribeygi, H., Maleki, M., Butler, A. E., Jamialahmadi, T., & Sahebkar, A. (2022). Molecular mechanisms linking stress and insulin resistance. EXCLI journal, 21, 317–334. https://doi.org/10.17179/excli2021-4382

Hackett, R. A., & Steptoe, A. (2017). Type 2 diabetes mellitus and psychological stress - a modifiable risk factor. Nature reviews. Endocrinology, 13(9), 547–560. https://doi.org/10.1038/nrendo.2017.64

"Sleep deprivation can impact..." (Page 100):
Briançon-Marjollet, A., Weiszenstein, M., Henri, M., Thomas, A., Godin-Ribuot, D., & Polak, J. (2015). The impact of sleep disorders on glucose metabolism: endocrine and molecular mechanisms. Diabetology & metabolic syndrome, 7, 25. https://doi.org/10.1186/s13098-015-0018-3

Antza, C., Kostopoulos, G., Mostafa, S., Nirantharakumar, K., & Tahrani, A. (2021). The links between sleep duration, obesity and type 2 diabetes mellitus. The Journal of endocrinology, 252(2), 125–141. https://doi.org/10.1530/JOE-21-0155

RECIPES

"...reduce insulin resistance." (Page 122):
Li, W., Ruan, W., Peng, Y., & Wang, D. (2018). Soy and the risk of type 2 diabetes mellitus: A systematic review and meta-analysis of observational studies. Diabetes research and clinical practice, 137, 190–199. https://doi.org/10.1016/j.diabres.2018.01.010

"...ginger may reduce blood sugar levels. (Page 133).
Ebrahimzadeh, A., Ebrahimzadeh, A., Mirghazanfari, S. M., Hazrati, E., Hadi, S., & Milajerdi, A. (2022). The effect of ginger supplementation on metabolic profiles in patients with type 2 diabetes mellitus: A systematic review and meta-analysis of randomized controlled trials. Complementary therapies in medicine, 65, 102802. https://doi.org/10.1016/j.ctim.2022.102802

"...improve blood sugar control and insulin sensitivity. (Page 134)

Viguiliouk E, Stewart SE, Jayalath VH, Ng AP, Mirrahimi A, de Souza RJ, Hanley AJ, Bazinet RP, Blanco Mejia S, Leiter LA, Josse RG, Kendall CW, Jenkins DJ, Sievenpiper JL. Effect of Replacing Animal Protein with Plant Protein on Glycemic Control in Diabetes: A Systematic Review and Meta-Analysis of Randomized Controlled Trials. Nutrients. 2015 Dec 1;7(12):9804-24. doi: 10.3390/nu7125509. PMID: 26633472; PMCID: PMC4690061.

"... reduce blood sugar levels and improve insulin resistance." (Page 145):
Anitha, S., Kane-Potaka, J., Tsusaka, T. W., Botha, R., Rajendran, A., Givens, D. I., Parasannanavar, D. J., Subramaniam, K., Prasad, K. D. V., Vetriventhan, M., & Bhandari, R. K. (2021). A Systematic Review and Meta-Analysis of the Potential of Millets for Managing and Reducing the Risk of Developing Diabetes Mellitus. Frontiers in nutrition, 8, 687428. https://doi.org/10.3389/fnut.2021.687428

"... improve insulin sensitivity (Page 153):
Viguiliouk E, Stewart SE, Jayalath VH, Ng AP, Mirrahimi A, de Souza RJ, Hanley AJ, Bazinet RP, Blanco Mejia S, Leiter LA, Josse RG, Kendall CW, Jenkins DJ, Sievenpiper JL. Effect of Replacing Animal Protein with Plant Protein on Glycemic Control in Diabetes: A Systematic Review and Meta-Analysis of Randomized Controlled Trials. Nutrients. 2015 Dec 1;7(12):9804-24. doi: 10.3390/nu7125509. PMID: 26633472; PMCID: PMC4690061.

"...consumption of soy is associated with..." (Page 161):
Li, W., Ruan, W., Peng, Y., & Wang, D. (2018). Soy and the risk of type 2 diabetes mellitus: A systematic review and meta-analysis of observational studies. Diabetes

research and clinical practice, 137, 190–199. https://doi.org/10.1016/j.diabres.2018.01.010

"Replacing red meat with plant-based proteins..." (Page 162):
Viguiliouk E, Stewart SE, Jayalath VH, Ng AP, Mirrahimi A, de Souza RJ, Hanley AJ, Bazinet RP, Blanco Mejia S, Leiter LA, Josse RG, Kendall CW, Jenkins DJ, Sievenpiper JL. Effect of Replacing Animal Protein with Plant Protein on Glycemic Control in Diabetes: A Systematic Review and Meta-Analysis of Randomized Controlled Trials. Nutrients. 2015 Dec 1;7(12):9804-24. doi: 10.3390/nu7125509. PMID: 26633472; PMCID: PMC4690061.

"Regular consumption of millet...." (Page 171):
Anitha, S., Kane-Potaka, J., Tsusaka, T. W., Botha, R., Rajendran, A., Givens, D. I., Parasannanavar, D. J., Subramaniam, K., Prasad, K. D. V., Vetriventhan, M., & Bhandari, R. K. (2021). A Systematic Review and Meta-Analysis of the Potential of Millets for Managing and Reducing the Risk of Developing Diabetes Mellitus. Frontiers in nutrition, 8, 687428. https://doi.org/10.3389/fnut.2021.687428

"Polyphenols may influence..." (Page 175)
Kim, Y., Keogh, J. B., & Clifton, P. M. (2016). Polyphenols and Glycemic Control. Nutrients, 8(1), 17. https://doi.org/10.3390/nu8010017

"...consuming an antioxidant-rich diet can help improve..." (Page 181)
Kim, Y., Keogh, J. B., & Clifton, P. M. (2016). Polyphenols and Glycemic Control. Nutrients, 8(1), 17. https://doi.org/10.3390/nu8010017

"Diets higher in magnesium..." (page 201):
Dubey, P., Thakur, V., & Chattopadhyay, M. (2020). Role of Minerals and Trace Elements in Diabetes and Insulin Resistance. Nutrients, 12(6), 1864. https://doi.org/10.3390/nu12061864

"...can help improve insulin resistance." (Page 210):
Vuksan V, Jenkins AL, Brissette C, Choleva L, Jovanovski E, Gibbs AL, Bazinet RP, Au-Yeung F, Zurbau A, Ho HV, Duvnjak L, Sievenpiper JL, Josse RG, Hanna A. Salba-chia (Salvia hispanica L.) in the treatment of overweight and obese patients with type 2 diabetes: A double-blind randomized controlled trial. Nutr Metab Cardiovasc Dis. 2017 Feb;27(2):138-146. doi: 10.1016/j.numecd.2016.11.124. Epub 2016 Dec 9. PMID: 28089080.

"...with lower risk of developing type 2 diabetes." (Page 213):
Muraki, I., Imamura, F., Manson, J. E., Hu, F. B., Willett, W. C., van Dam, R. M., & Sun, Q. (2013). Fruit consumption and risk of type 2 diabetes: results from three prospective longitudinal cohort studies. BMJ (Clinical research ed.), 347, f5001. https://doi.org/10.1136/bmj.f5001

"Eating polyphenol-rich foods is associated with..." (Page 214):
Kim, Y., Keogh, J. B., & Clifton, P. M. (2016). Polyphenols and Glycemic Control. Nutrients, 8(1), 17. https://doi.org/10.3390/nu8010017

"...the polyphenols in cacao may help... (Page 216)
Kim, Y., Keogh, J. B., & Clifton, P. M. (2016). Polyphenols and Glycemic Control. Nutrients, 8(1), 17. https://doi.org/10.3390/nu8010017

"...consumption of walnuts is associated with..." (Page 222):
Pan, A., Sun, Q., Manson, J. E., Willett, W. C., & Hu, F. B. (2013). Walnut consumption is associated with lower risk of type 2 diabetes in women. The Journal of nutrition, 143(4), 512–518. https://doi.org/10.3945/jn.112.172171

"...zinc influences insulin functioning..." Page 231:
Dubey, P., Thakur, V., & Chattopadhyay, M. (2020). Role of Minerals and Trace Elements in Diabetes and Insulin Resistance. Nutrients, 12(6), 1864. https://doi.org/10.3390/nu12061864

"... selenium Brazil nuts in the diet..." (Page 239):
Ouyang, J., Cai, Y., Song, Y., Gao, Z., Bai, R., & Wang, A. (2022). Potential Benefits of Selenium Supplementation in Reducing Insulin Resistance in Patients with Cardiometabolic Diseases: A Systematic Review and Meta-Analysis. Nutrients, 14(22), 4933. https://doi.org/10.3390/nu14224933

"...help improve insulin resistance." (Page 243):
Jackson, C. L., & Hu, F. B. (2014). Long-term associations of nut consumption with body weight and obesity. The American journal of clinical nutrition, 100 Suppl 1(1), 408S–11S. https://doi.org/10.3945/ajcn.113.071332

"... may also help with reducing insulin resistance." (Page 247):
Takahashi, F., Hashimoto, Y., Kaji, A., Sakai, R., Miki, A., Okamura, T., Kitagawa, N., Okada, H., Nakanishi, N., Majima, S., Senmaru, T., Ushigome, E., Hamaguchi, M., Asano, M., Yamazaki, M., & Fukui, M. (2021). Habitual Miso (Fermented Soybean Paste) Consumption Is Associated with Glycemic Variability in Patients with Type 2 Diabetes: A Cross-Sectional Study. Nutrients, 13(5), 1488. https://doi.org/10.3390/nu13051488

Index

Page numbers in *italics* refer to figures.

Acknowledgments

While there may be times when there are "too many cooks in the kitchen," the preparation of this book was not one of them! A prodigious amount of work was required, and a prodigious effort was given by so many, including:

Cristina García and Margarita Marcelino: thank you for your tireless work supporting us in the kitchen. Your top-notch culinary skills and impeccable taste buds helped transform these recipes into nutritious works of art. If there's one person who knows the recipes better than us, it's Cristina. Her passion for plant-based cooking and her innate cooking skills dazzled everyone around her.

Bob Licalzi and Diane Maldonado: thank you for letting us turn their beautiful kitchen into our workspace. Diane, thank you for being our master taste tester; her standard became our benchmark for the book — if a recipe didn't make it past her discerning palate, then it was back to the kitchen. Bob, you have a gift with words; thank you for providing your editing skills and helping us make our book more engaging.

Everyone at our phenomenal team at Reversing T2D, including Dr. Sandra Sobel, Amy Brownstein, Cara Berger, Lauren Ranley, Xavier Toledo, Gia Padula, and Nisreen Shumayrikh.

Sandra, thank you for your mentorship and always being so willing to share your expertise and guidance; Amy, for going above and beyond to support us with anything we needed; and Nisreen, for helping us include more diverse recipes.

Our photography team: Robert Alvarez, Andrea Pérez, and Cristina Cardona. Robert, you completely blew us away with your photography skills. You were such a pleasure to work with and we couldn't have thought of a better person for the job. Andrea, you were born to direct! Thank you for your direction and guidance throughout the photoshoot. Cristina, you have a gift for food styling. We hope you bestow that gift on many others.

Peter and Brenna Licalzi, Lindsay Wilkes-Edrington, Megan Kesting, Christine McKnight, and the rest of the team at Blue Star Press. Thank you, Peter, for giving us this opportunity and believing in our vision. Brenna, we are in awe of your drive and work ethic. Thank you for seeing our potential and doing everything in your power to ensure the book's success. To Lindsay, for handling every logistical aspect in the creation of this book and being so amenable to all our requests to push back our deadlines. Megan, we are mesmerized by your design talent and giving life to our book, and Christine, your editing skills are unparalleled.

Individually, Diana would like to thank the following people:

My mother, Diane Maldonado, for her endless support, encouragement, attention to detail, and her willingness to always go above and beyond; my father, Bob Licalzi, and his contribution to sustainability by never letting a single crumb of food go to waste; my husband, Andrew Pettersen, for never once doubting my ability to juggle being a new mom and write a cookbook and for always being my rock; Ruth Bader Ginsburg for her inspiring post-partum story, motivating me to "pick myself up and find a way"; and of course, my business partner, Jose Tejero, for believing in my abilities and direction for this book.

Individually, Jose would like to thank:

My mother, Gladys Del Pozo, for her everlasting support and assurance that anything I believe in can be achieved; my girlfriend, Kelley Johnson, for her encouragement and unmatched cooking skills; and my business partner, Diana Licalzi, for having the vision for this cookbook and executing it flawlessly.

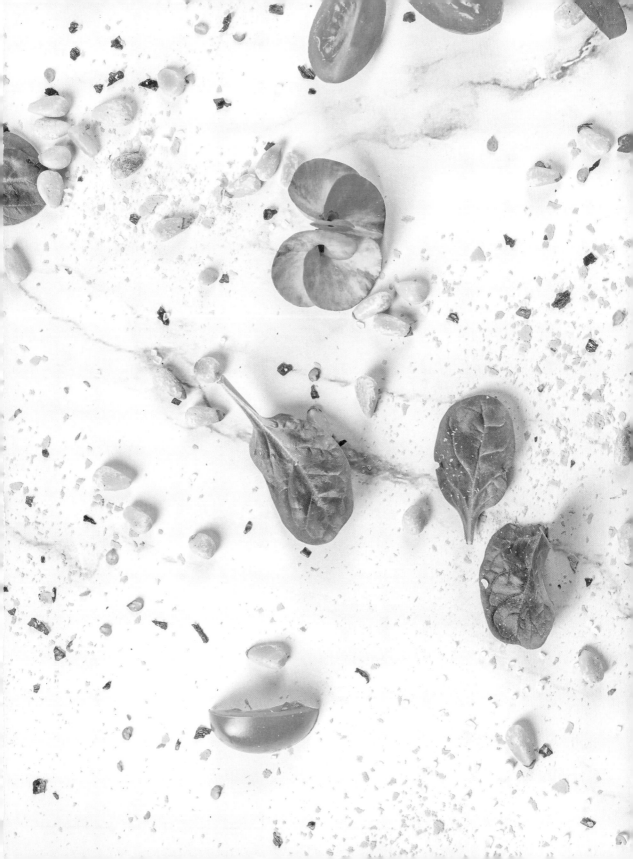

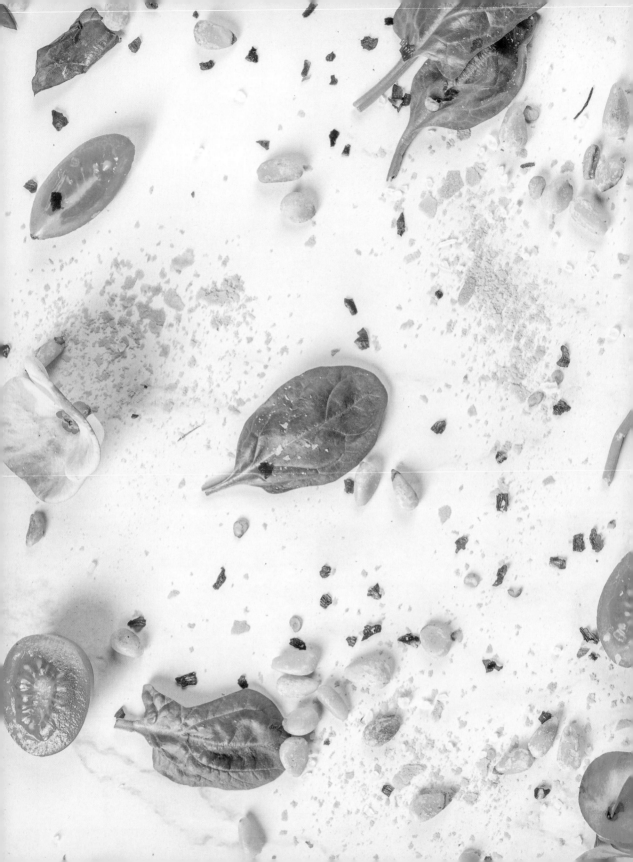